GW00832252

Forgive Me For Not Shaking Hands

Forgive Me For Not Shaking Hands

To Lisa

Best wishes

Love

Forgive Me for Not Shaking Hands

The story of a child excluded from school for wearing a splint

Barbara Blackston Huntley

Forgive Me For Not Shaking Hands

First published in Great Britain in 2014 by Rodney House

Second Edition published in Great Britain 2015 by Rodney House

Email: b.blackstonhuntley@gmail.com

ISBN: 978-0-9930400-0-9

Printed by Book Printing UK
Remus House, Coltsfoot Drive, Peterborough, PE2 9BF

ACKNOWLEDGEMENTS

My thanks to Vicki Prescott, who typed up some of my early manuscript, and to all those people who read it and offered their comments.

My thanks also to Dinks for her design input and to Mike Truscott whose comments helped me more than he knows.

FOREWORD

Forgive Me for Not Shaking Hands is an autobiography, written originally for my grandchildren, and also to record the effects of polio, which is a disease I hope will have been eradicated by the time they are my age.

In addition, I would like to think that in some way it might help to raise a contribution for the British Polio Fellowship listed at the end of the book.

It is also a record of a working class family from the 1930s to the early years of the 21st Century. None of this family who were born before the 1980s were famous, well educated or achieved outstanding careers or performed feats of daring adventure.

So why did I write this book, you may ask. I just felt I had to record my world before it and I were gone forever.

I would like to think that my grandchildren might find the time and energy to write about their own lives one day – and that these stories could then be gathered alongside mine so that readers of the future can have permanent access to an interesting chronicle of family life now and in the past.

The famous and infamous are frequently written about, but it is mostly 'ordinary' people, who lead unrecorded lives, who have made our country what it is today!

Barbara Blackston Huntley, 01 May 2014

NB: After the death of Rodney Blackston in 2005 Barbara married Ralph Huntley in 2008.

by Barbara Blackston Huntley

CHAPTER ONE

POLIO STRIKES

The shattering of my much-loved, rather delicate blue teacup, as it fell out of my hand and onto the floor, was the moment my mother was left in no doubt that something was terribly wrong. Then my hallucinations – seeing**, scary** faces at my upstairs bedroom window – drove her to contact our doctor urgently. The doctor, in turn, told her to send immediately for my father, who was away on a training course for his job. My father cried at the news when he returned, something I had never seen him do before in my short life.

I was two months short of my fifth birthday – but my life, and the lives of my parents, had just changed forever. The shocking transformation began with a seven-week separation. I was sent to an isolation sanatorium and was not allowed to see them once in that time – and worse, nobody told me why. Little wonder that I feared I had been abandoned.

Hitler was doing his worst and Britain was embroiled in history's greatest global conflict, but this – the nightmare upheaval of our lives triggered by my inability to lift a teacup – is my dominant memory from those early 1940s years.

The excitement of the year I was born, 1937, had been the coronation of George VI after his brother's abdication the year before. For my parents, the excitement had been managing a holiday in the Isle of Wight and, no doubt, my birth. Alas, there were to be no more holidays for quite a while.

I grew up in Erith in Kent. Looking back, I always think of my home as being warm, cosy and secure and of my mother as always being industrious and fussing around my father and me. I adored my father, as he did me; his health was not good and he had always to be careful as he had ankylosing spondylitis (a bone and muscle disease of the spine) and duodenal ulcers. He always let me sit on his lap for a cuddle before going to bed and I would comb his hair or persuade him to read me a story. He always had the biggest chair in the room. It had big wooden arms and I could sit on them, making them very shiny over the years; I loved the feel of them. When I was ill, the chair would be made into a bed, which I thought was great fun, and sometimes my mother would sleep downstairs, too, if I was very ill and needed to stay in a warm room.

We also had a telephone - a very rare commodity in the 1930s and 40s for an ordinary working class family. My father was a telephone engineer, but he did not get his telephone free, contrary to what all the neighbours seemed to think (much to my mother's chagrin) because he was employed by the GPO. Everyone in the neighbourhood used our phone to call the doctor or to pass on messages of death, illness or being kept late at work. Our meals were frequently interrupted by this message passing and my mother was convinced people waited to drop dead until we were eating!

My early memories relate to World War II on the home front. One night I woke up, when sleeping in the Anderson Shelter at the bottom of the garden, during an air raid to hear my mother screaming dreadfully. This was very frightening; however, the cause was not a bomb but a small spider, which had the audacity to crawl into my mother's ear, causing her to become hysterical. The neighbours gathered round after the 'all-clear' siren had sounded, thinking my mother had been injured, but the only first aid she needed was given by my father. He had the good sense to shine a torch into her ear, which caused the spider to crawl out towards the warmth! After that, we always laid in our bunks wearing rubber earplugs and scarves tightly tied around our heads.

Two months before my fifth birthday, I had to be vaccinated for diphtheria, which was a common disease that had killed many children at that time. I was taken to the local children's clinic and lined up with many other children for my jab. My right arm was quite sore during the days following and I developed a sore throat. My parents noticed I was not using my arm very much and eventually called the doctor. He said I had tonsillitis, collected his half crown (12½p) fee and went on his way.

But from then on my condition deteriorated rapidly – climaxing with that never-to-be-forgotten morning when I told my mother I could not pick up that cup I was so fond of. 'Don't be silly, pick it up properly!' she said. The shattering outcome convinced her that there was something more than tonsillitis ailing me. Money for doctor's fees was not easy to find from my father's income, so first of all I was put to bed. My temperature and headache became worse, though, followed first by those hallucinations and then, within just a few hours, an inability to stand. My grandmother, who lived next door to us, told my mother to call the doctor quickly as she thought I had meningitis.

The doctor examined me and began to realise that I was seriously ill. My beloved Daddy returned home as quickly as public transport would allow; he was devastated by what had happened and I can still see so clearly his tearful face reflected in a mirror over the fireplace in my bedroom. Our family GP called another doctor - an ex-army man who had seen many cases of polio. He confirmed that I had what was then known as Infantile Paralysis but is now called Polio. There was little or no medication available to treat polio victims; it is a virus – I have Spinal Polio which attacked the motor neurons in my spinal cord. It can cause paralysis in arms and legs and breathing problems.

I had to be sent to an isolation hospital where no contact with my parents would be permitted. An ambulance was arranged, and I remember my mother asking what I would like for my tea before it came! 'Can I have a tomato to eat like an apple?' I replied.

When the ambulance arrived, my parents were told they could not even kiss me goodbye because of the extent of the infection, but I think they did anyway; polio could be passed on during the original infection by mouth to mouth contact or in the faeces. Children under five years were particularly susceptible, hence the original name of Infantile Paralysis; however anyone could be infected. Many homes were fumigated when a member of the family caught Polio.

Although they were not allowed to visit me, my mother and father wrote letters - but my problem was that I had not yet learnt to read. So a nurse would read their letter to me, take it away to be destroyed. Even the Teddy Bear I had taken into hospital could not accompany me when I left that first hospital. I assume it too had to be destroyed.

By now I was paralysed all down my right side. Two other girls shared my isolation; we had all caught the disease around the same time. After seven weeks, when the infection had subsided, I was moved to West Hill Hospital in Dartford, a major general hospital at the time. My mother was told that I was to be transferred and she was permitted to visit on Wednesday and Sunday afternoons for two hours only. No other visits were normally allowed unless patients were expected to die.

My mother and grandmother immediately went to the hospital and as they got to the gates an ambulance pulled in and stopped. My mother asked if it was her daughter in the ambulance; the driver said it was and he allowed them to see me for a few minutes. As the doors opened, there were Mummy and Grandma smiling broadly – only for their faces to turn to a look of shock that mystified me. Many years later, my mother explained that I was almost unrecognisable as the healthy, happy four-year-old of two months earlier. Polio had taken its terrifying toll.

My new home for the next seven months was a large open ward. The bed had a black iron frame and my right arm was tied with a bandage to the rail of the bed head. What this treatment was supposed to achieve, I never had any idea. In fact, I believe that, and the later splinting, contributed to the lifelong deformity of my arm. The nursing staff were generally kindly but very strict in keeping to hospital rules and I soon became very institutionalised. An enamel mug of tea at dawn woke us each day and mealtimes were rigorously held at the same time each day, ending with an enamel mug of cocoa at bedtime.

As well as coping with patients' standard needs, the staff also encountered many problems from the constant air raids as this was during the London Baedeker raids of wartime Britain in 1942; the Germans were bombing very heavily from Dover to

London. The hospital was in 'bomb alley' - less than 20 miles from London and close to railway lines and the River Thames,

I recall no fear then - just the hustle and bustle before and after air raids. The nurses would pull the heads of two cots together, with one sitting in the 'V' between the two little patients. An enamel bowl was placed over each face as a protection from flying shrapnel; a pillow covered this. I used to think it was all a rather funny game. When a bomb exploded close to my hospital ward, a lot of shrapnel came through the ceiling and went straight through the floor and (thankfully) an empty bed! Fortunately, no-one was seriously hurt, but I remember the soldiers in their tin helmets coming into the ward carrying hurricane lamps, as there were no lights. Unaware of the cause or consequence of war, I found this very exciting.

Because of the restrictions on the parental visits, there was little else to look forward to. We were not allowed our tea until visitors had left the ward. I was always hungry, so I used to encourage my family to go home promptly, which must have hurt my mother no end!

I remember the fantastic Christmas we had there. A huge Christmas tree, so tall that the top had to be removed, was brought into the ward. How they managed to get the tree in wartime, I have no idea, but as I had never seen one before I was absolutely amazed. I have never forgotten the thrill of receiving two presents from that tree - a black doll and some doll's house furniture. That night we had green jelly for tea - a real treat - with bread and jam being the normal teatime fare! I thought it was wonderful and to this day the sight of green jelly makes me feel happy.

A not so happy memory of food was the day I refused to eat my greens; I hated the waterlogged dollops of mush that we were served, but on this occasion I was going to endure a torture that also has never been forgotten. Along came a redheaded nurse who would have been better employed by the Gestapo. If it was the last thing she did, she was going to make me eat that plate of greens and for two hours she forced the now cold food into my heaving mouth. It was to warp my view of greens and redheads for many years!

Meanwhile, I had to learn to walk again; the paralysis had subsided from my right leg, but the muscles were much weakened and at first it was difficult to stand. Time and effort by the staff gradually brought back enough strength for me to take my first tottery steps. The fingers of my right hand began to recover some movement. However, the muscle which pulls the thumb up and the muscles of the upper arm and shoulder were never to work again and eventually shrivelled up. When I became adult, this arm was about five inches (130 mm) shorter than the left one. The arm hung loose from the shoulder socket when not splinted and the hand was turned outward with my thumb stuck out and my fingers curled. People these days are kept better informed about their illnesses. I assumed my arm would one day be normal again. The realisation that it wouldn't was very gradual and I sometimes wonder if maybe this was not a better way of coming to terms with a permanent disability.

I finally went back home to my parents, wearing a very heavy plaster cast all over my back from bottom to neck and up my paralysed arm, after those seven months in hospital. I was always an only child, but my mother came from a big family. Aunts, uncles and cousins lived nearby, along with my maternal grandmother in the house next door and my paternal grandparents across the road. A large box awaited my return. I opened it excitedly and found a 'big dolly,' as she was always called; it was the size of a real baby. My family had managed to buy her second-hand and my mother had made her a new set of clothes out of her old clothes. I could not believe my eyes. I loved her dearly on sight!

During the last year of the war, I become a very nervous little girl. Because of the constant bombing, it seemed as if I were spending all my life in our air-raid shelter, which was made of corrugated iron and half-buried in our back garden. It smelled of damp earth and paraffin. The latter was used for the little stove which was our heating and also the means by which we boiled our little tin kettle for cups of tea.

My father rigged a little bell with batteries to warn the neighbours when I saw approaching aeroplanes or 'doodlebugs' (German unmanned rockets) coming overhead. I could spot them from where I sat in the doorway of the shelter - too frightened to go indoors even when the all-clear siren had sounded. When my bell rang, Mother would run down the garden to see what was worrying me; if the siren went, we shut ourselves in the shelter until we heard the all-clear siren signalling the end of an air raid. My mother would then return to the house to continue her housework or cooking if it was daytime. If the weather was fine, the local housewives would gather their children about them and get together with their neighbours. They sat near a shelter where they could knit socks and pullovers for their men folk who were away fighting. Or they would repair the clothes and bedding that could not be replaced because of rationing and the need to make do and mend. The conversation usually revolved around worries about their husbands and the lack of food or who had 'copped it' in the air raid the night before.

A raid that went into our family folklore came just as my mother had finished cooking rissoles, one of my father's favourite meals. Carrying his meal on a plate, she ran down the garden to the air raid shelter, which had a little shelf that my father used as a table. He had hardly picked up his knife and fork when a bomb blast covered his rissoles! The day 'father lost his rissoles in the war' became an enduring family joke!

During this time, my mother had to take me to see the consultant at West Hill Hospital, Dartford regularly. This was often an all day trip waiting to be seen sitting on hard chairs in dreary waiting rooms with no special facilities or toys for children. My mother took pencils, paper, little books and a sandwich for our lunch and I clasped my black dolly in my left arm. She also had to take me to a local cottage hospital in Erith three times a week for treatment to my right arm, left paralysed by the polio. A physiotherapist there was very kind to me and I liked him very much; he made me laugh a lot while he fitted electrodes to my arm, which he then placed in a small bath of water, switching on the current. I used to grit my teeth then, as it was so painful. I think it was called Faradayism; Michael Faraday had discovered electrical impulses could stimulate the muscles to work again. Unfortunately it did not work for me. This was followed by exercises and massage, which I found very comforting. By this time the plaster cast had been removed and I had to wear a splint on my arm, paid for by my parents. I have a letter dated April 15, 1943, asking for the sum of £2.10s for one splint. This was a considerable sum then, probably representing almost a week's earnings for my father. The NHS did not exist then so all splints for arms and callipers worn on legs had to be paid for in advance of the items being made.

When Christmas came, my physiotherapist gave me a lovely rag doll. I thought her the loveliest thing I had ever seen; she had flaming red plaits and wore a green velvet suit. A game I played with my dolls was to give them electrical treatment using jelly moulds for the bath of imaginary water and bits of fuse wire bound to their arms for the electricity!

My parents became concerned for my mental well-being as the air raids were continuing to make me very nervous. I had many nightmares about bombs and was afraid my whole family would be killed. One night a bomb dropped in a field behind the houses on the other side of the road from our house; it blew all the windows out and the doors off their hinges in our house and some of the houses on the other side of the road. It cracked our bedroom walls, although they did not fall down. My parents and me were at this time sleeping indoors under an iron table called a Morrison shelter; it was like a double bed with an iron roof and legs about the height of a dining room table. The sides were made of strong horizontal and vertical wires and when you got inside they were fixed to the sides to stop the large debris from injuring the occupants. The noise of the air raid was deafening and as I lay between my parents we clung together and were very frightened. I remember my mother saying to my father 'this is our lot, Ern!' but the raid ended and the dust settled.

For the sake of my own mental health, she and Dad decided that I should be evacuated. However, my polio stopped me from going under the normal government scheme. My mother had to find someone who was prepared to take me in privately, with her accompanying me, because of the constant hospital treatment I needed. Through the WVS (later the WRVS - Women's Royal Voluntary Service), she made contact with a lady in Yorkshire who was prepared to take my mother and me.

by Barbara Blackston Huntley

My mother did not want to leave my father, especially as he was in such poor health and working underground in the telephone exchanges. It was essential to repair damaged lines quickly to ensure that emergency calls could be dealt with as fast as possible (long before the computer age).

When all was arranged for my evacuation, my mother and I bid a tearful farewell to my father and went by train to Yorkshire. I had never been so far before or seen so much; it was a very exciting journey for a six-year-old who had never travelled. The train was packed with evacuees and soldiers who sat on kit bags. They told me stories and showed me things out of the windows - things that I had never seen before, such as cows and sheep and high hills. I suppose I was spoilt more than other children because I wore a splint on my arm, which was stuck up in the air at right angles to my body. It looked as if I was permanently asking to be excused! (The plaster and splints I had as a child are now in the Science Museum in South Kensington, London). The back plaster I wore before and after leaving hospital was shown in the film "The Battle to Beat Polio" shown on BBC2 in May 2014.

.

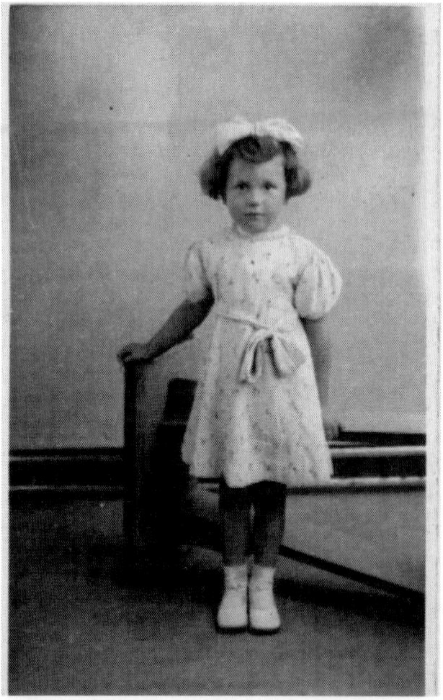

Barbara shortly before she caught the polio virus in 1942.

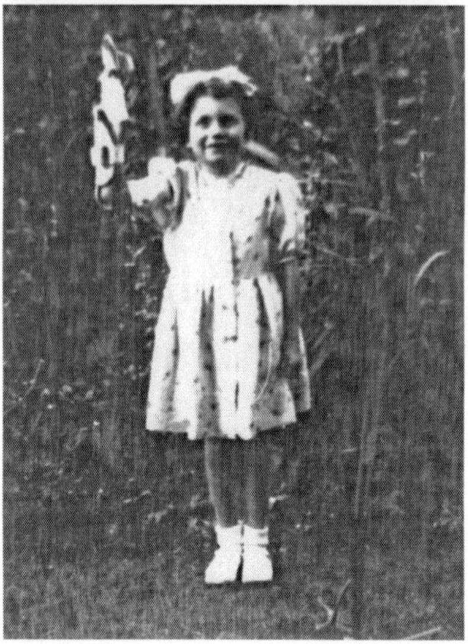

The splinted arm worn day & night. Aged 6.

CHAPTER TWO

EVACUATION

Whatever else you could say about my childhood, the one thing it was NOT was uneventful! First, there was the devastating upheaval wrought by my polio; then it was all change once more as an evacuee. We – my mother and I – were made to feel both welcome and unwelcome at the bungalow where we first stayed in Redburn Avenue in Shipley, Yorkshire. The man of the house made little effort to hide his dissatisfaction with our presence, but his wife was very kind to us. Oh, and my new friendship with a local owl also helped!

Mrs Campbell was a young voluntary nurse in a local hospital, the daughter of a local doctor; she was vivacious and friendly, married to a much older and very serious businessman. My mother and I were considered to be of a much lower class than him. However, provided we stayed in the kitchen, or our bedroom, and did not venture into the lounge or dining room, we were tolerated well enough. Mrs Campbell would eat with us when her husband was not at home and she and my mother got on very well together. She owned a lovely shiny black cat called Mickey, but I was once told off by Mrs Campbell for kicking poor Mickey after losing my temper (the only time I remember doing so)! I felt very ashamed of my action and feared that she would no longer be friendly towards me, but I need not have worried.

The owl, which I named Tony, would fly in through the kitchen window at dawn from a great big tree at the back of the house. Perching on the high kitchen mantelpiece, he would be given leftover scraps of food; he particularly liked a bacon rind. After his breakfast, he flew back to the tree, presumably to sleep all day. I was very fond of Tony as I had never had a pet before. Alas, one morning Tony went to perch on a jug of milk standing on the mantelpiece. He sent it flying, with the milk spewing everywhere and smashing the jug. After that, he was strictly banned from the house and the loss of my first pet was very painful.

Mrs Campbell loved her voluntary nursing work, helping the wounded soldiers back from the front, and she was very kind to me when I caught diphtheria. This was a very serious illness then, often fatal. I had been vaccinated, which probably gave me more chance of recovery, although it was after the vaccination that I had contracted polio. So once more I went into isolation, this time at Keighley Hospital, for a month. I was not allowed visitors because of the infection risk, a fact that once more no-one explained to me. So once again, as a very frightened young child, I thought I had been deserted. Children's thoughts and feelings were rarely considered in those days and often they had to face very frightening things alone because they were regarded as too young to understand. I recall intense fear of many medical procedures, but I always said nothing because I did not know how to express such fears.

When I could get up, some of the wounded soldiers were allowed to walk me round the grounds. One sat me on his lap on a seat in the grounds, telling me about his own little girl at home and how he missed her very much. I felt he was my "special friend" when everyone else had gone away and left me; he often waved to me through the windows when I couldn't go out.

At Christmas, my father was able to come up to Yorkshire. We were invited by Mrs Campbell's father, Dr Hayes-Smith, and his wife, to spend the holiday in their home while they were away. The reason for their absence, tragically, was the death of their only son on active service. They were so desolate at his loss that they felt they could not stay in their lovely home. I suppose really it was a typical middle class home of the 1940s, but to me it was a magical place. There was a soft rug to sit on in front of the fire, red tiles on the kitchen floor and a pale blue bedroom with large mahogany wardrobes and twin beds with very shiny head and foot boards - much softer beds than my hard flock mattress at home. There were lots of books and a big squishy sofa in the lounge; It was wonderful to have 'Mummy and Daddy' together with me. I still have a small book of 'Cinderella' with beautiful coloured pictures that Mrs Campbell gave me. I loved that book and think it was my first romantic ideal. I also had a big book (all in black and white) of nursery rhymes. Both these books gave many hours of pleasure and were much treasured possessions.

Unknown to me, Mr and Mrs Campbell's marriage was not working out and he remained unhappy at having my mother and me staying in the house. He decided that we must leave and we were transferred to a new billet. This was such a contrast to the comfort we had enjoyed in Redburn Avenue. It was a house that had been rented to the army by the owners. The army had not taken care of it and after they left it was occupied by a pregnant woman and her three children, her husband being a soldier and away.

We had to share with the family already living there and we found the house very bare, dirty and smelly. We had few possessions, so life was bleak. My mother and I had one room to ourselves and shared an attic bedroom. We were given two folding chairs, one dining table, two camp beds, two knives, forks, teaspoons, one teapot, two cups, saucers, tea plates and dinner plates. We had dark grey army blankets and straw filled pillows covered in grey striped ticking, but there were no sheets or pillowcases and no armchairs. My father eventually sent our sheets from home, but there were very few comforts and I was often ill. I was lucky enough to be treated by Dr Hayes-Smith, who did not charge my mother. This was before the National Health Service and all doctors normally had to be paid unless you were a member of their panel, in which case an amount was paid weekly as a kind of medical insurance. However, it was generally only the doctors who worked with the poor who ran such schemes and Dr Hayes-Smith was not one of those.

I would cry at night, missing my Daddy and all my extended family at home. I was also frightened of the very cold, dark attic bedroom, with just a tiny window high in the roof that rattled when it was windy. Appropriately, the place was called Windhill. The grey blankets made my skin itch and the straw pillows were hard and uncomfortable. Our unhygienic conditions must have been the cause of our getting scabies - small insects that burrow under the skin and cause irritation. The cure was to take frequent very unpleasant smelling sulphur baths.

Our stay in the billet was made much easier by the family next door - an elderly couple, their son and his wife and daughter. They were typical down-to-earth Yorkshire folk with accents much broader than those of today. At first I could hardly understand them, but as time went on my speech imitated theirs, much to the amusement of my relatives when I returned home. I was teased unmercifully for saying things like 'We got on a buzz (bus)' and 'I am having a bath' (rhyming with Cath rather than 'barth,' as it is pronounced in the south). But while evacuated I was always referred to as the 'Little Cockney Girl'.

I was only months away from my seventh birthday when we were evacuated, but I had still not been to school apart from about three months in the infants. There were no special schools in Kent for disabled children and the state schools were very reluctant to admit me; they felt the strange splint on my arm would be a distraction for other children and they did not want the responsibility of anything going wrong. In my brief stay in the local infant school at Brook Street in Erith, I was made to feel very odd and different from the other children. I was not allowed to use scissors or go out to play in the playground for fear of hurting myself! I had longed to join in the games with the others and I was allowed to use scissors at home, so I could not understand why things were different at school. How attitudes have changed since then; such a situation would be unthinkable now, when all sorts of disabilities in children are accepted and integrated into ordinary schools, although prejudice persists in many areas.

The authorities in Yorkshire in 1944 appeared to be much more enlightened than those in Kent and had a very different attitude to those with special educational needs. I will always be grateful to those who recognised my needs and made every effort to educate me at a very difficult time in our history. I was sent to a special school for disabled children – Lister Lane School, Bradford which is now closed. I was encouraged to do everything myself, receive a normal education, and in addition was given treatment for my arm. I was happy there and made some good friends.

While evacuated, my mother took me to the cinema for the first time. I was amazed; I stared and stared at this giant silver screen with the "moving, talking pictures." Remember, these were the days before ordinary homes had TV. I forget what the film was, but there was a scene with girls dancing in full-skirted dresses, filmed from above their heads as they swirled round and round. I couldn't believe my eyes; it was so pretty and so far removed from my make-do and mend world. Only one other film stands in my memory as a child and that was 'Scott of the Antarctic'. I became so involved in the story that when Captain Oates walked out of the tent to his death I cried out loud and had to be removed from the cinema!

We returned home at the end of the war on Tuesday, June 12, 1945. As the train trundled through London, I was horrified at the sight of all the bombed buildings, the shattered homes of so many. Some walls were intact with rubble all around them, but my dominant thought was that I was going home to my beloved Daddy and to the large family of relations who at that time all lived around us.

Our home had suffered bomb damage. Ceilings had collapsed and windows had been blown in, but these had been patched up by the time we returned. I burst into tears when I saw how my doll's pram and big doll had been damaged; the pram lining had been shredded by the blast and the doll badly scratched and her clothes torn. She was my special doll who had been waiting for me when I returned from hospital. Although neither she nor the pram was anywhere near new, to me they were the best things I had ever had. However, things were soon put back to rights and the bomb damage men soon came to repair the house.

While my parents were clearing up after the repair men, I went to play in the garden and saw two cats having a fight. In my rush to separate them, I tripped and my splinted right arm went snap. The hospital diagnosed a green stick fracture and my arm was put in plaster with a sling, which I must say made a change from being stuck up in the air! It was very painful being put in a different position at the same time as the fracture.

This episode was the last that comes to mind from my war years, but some 40 years later there was a sequel to our stay in Mr and Mrs Campbell's bungalow. In 1984 my mother traced the former Mrs Campbell, she was now Mrs Drummond living in Kent. We met and I was able to give her some flowers to say thank you for helping us through the first months of evacuation.

by Barbara Blackston Huntley

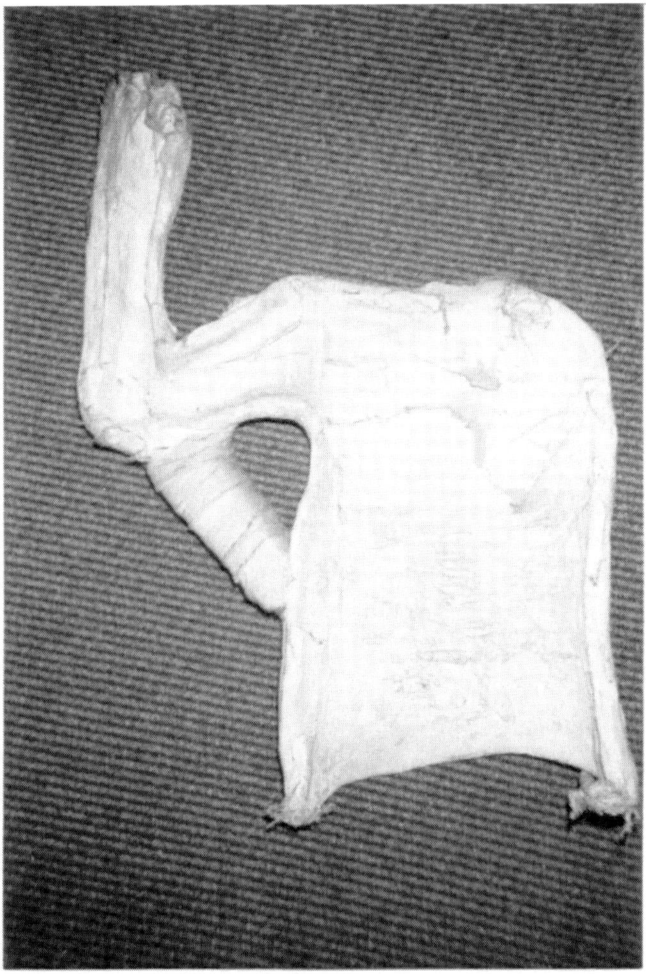

First Plaster Cast worn aged 5 years, now in the Science Museum.

It was shown in the film "The Battle to Beat Polio"

Broadcast in May 2014.

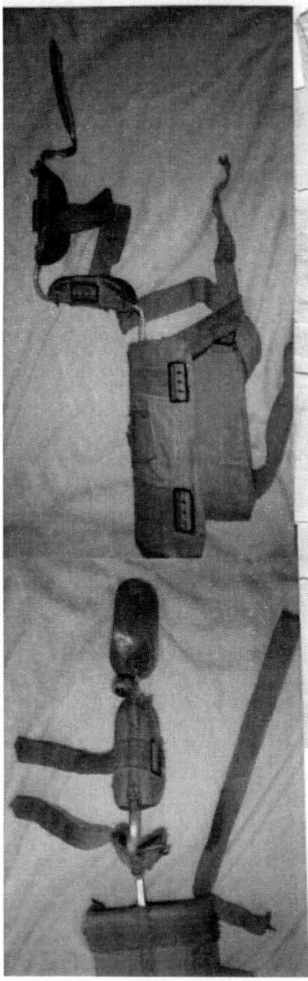

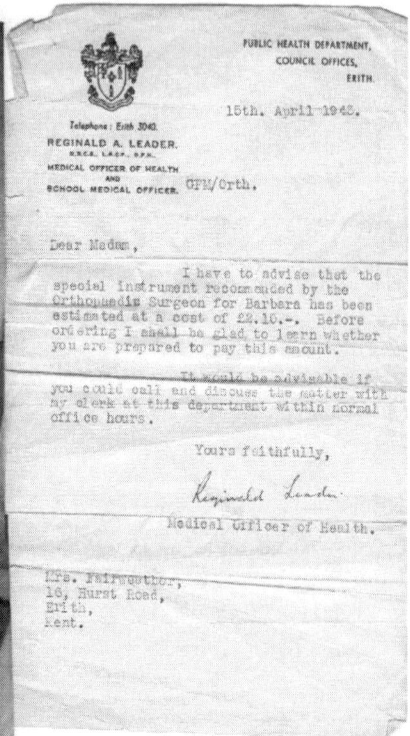

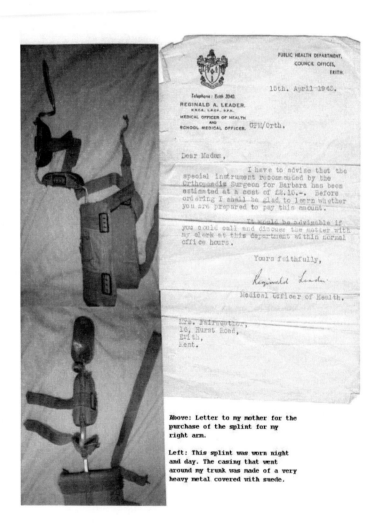

PUBLIC HEALTH DEPARTMENT,
COUNCIL OFFICES,
ERITH.

Telephone: Erith 3040.
REGINALD A. LEADER.
M.R.C.S., L.R.C.P., D.P.H.
MEDICAL OFFICER OF HEALTH
AND
SCHOOL MEDICAL OFFICER.

15th. April 1943.

GFM/Orth.

Dear Madam,

I have to advise that the special instrument recommended by the Orthopaedic Surgeon for Barbara has been estimated at a cost of £2.10.-. Before ordering I shall be glad to learn whether you are prepared to pay this amount.

It would be advisable if you could call and discuss the matter with my clerk at this department within normal office hours.

Yours faithfully,

Reginald Leader

Medical Officer of Health.

Mrs. Fairweather,
16, Hurst Road,
Erith,
Kent.

Above: Letter to my mother for the purchase of the splint for my right arm.

Left: This splint was worn night and day. The casing that went around my trunk was made of a very heavy metal covered with suede.

by Barbara Blackston Huntley

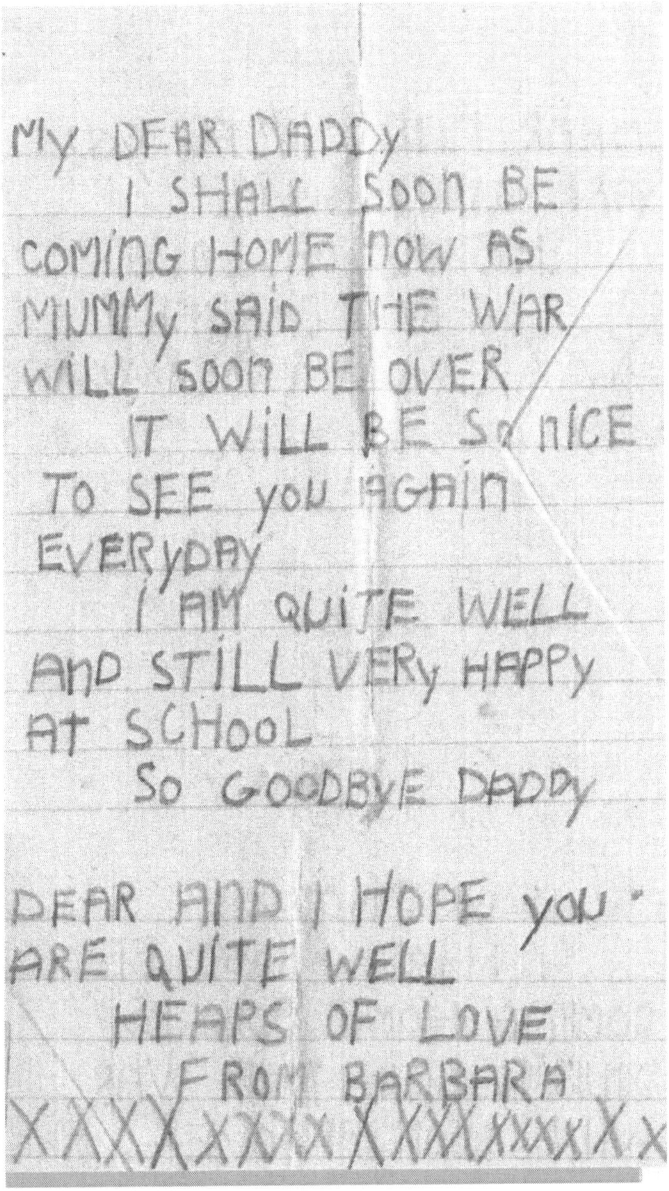

MY DEAR DADDY
I SHALL SOON BE
COMING HOME NOW AS
MUMMY SAID THE WAR
WILL SOON BE OVER
IT WILL BE SO NICE
TO SEE YOU AGAIN
EVERYDAY
I AM QUITE WELL
AND STILL VERY HAPPY
AT SCHOOL
SO GOODBYE DADDY

DEAR AND I HOPE YOU
ARE QUITE WELL
HEAPS OF LOVE
FROM BARBARA
XXXXXXXXXXXXXXXXXXX

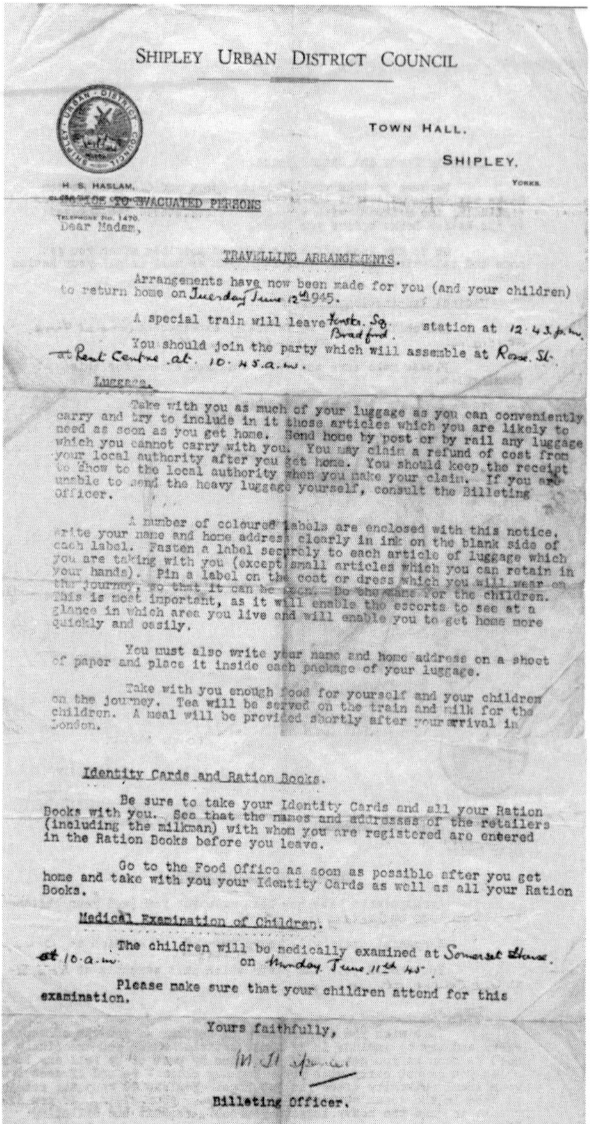

SHIPLEY URBAN DISTRICT COUNCIL

TOWN HALL.

SHIPLEY.

YORKS.

H. S. HASLAM,

NOTICE TO EVACUATED PERSONS

TELEPHONE No. 1470.

Dear Madam,

TRAVELLING ARRANGEMENTS.

Arrangements have now been made for you (and your children) to return home on Tuesday June 12th 1945.

A special train will leave Forster Sq. Bradford. station at 12.43 p.m.

You should join the party which will assemble at Rose St. Rest Centre at 10.45 a.m.

Luggage.

Take with you as much of your luggage as you can conveniently carry and try to include in it those articles which you are likely to need as soon as you get home. Send home by post or by rail any luggage which you cannot carry with you. You may claim a refund of cost from your local authority after you get home. You should keep the receipt to show to the local authority when you make your claim. If you are unable to send the heavy luggage yourself, consult the Billeting Officer.

A number of coloured labels are enclosed with this notice. Write your name and home address clearly in ink on the blank side of each label. Fasten a label securely to each article of luggage which you are taking with you (except small articles which you can retain in your hands). Pin a label on the coat or dress which you will wear on the journey, so that it can be seen. Do the same for the children. This is most important, as it will enable the escorts to see at a glance in which area you live and will enable you to get home more quickly and easily.

You must also write your name and home address on a sheet of paper and place it inside each package of your luggage.

Take with you enough food for yourself and your children on the journey. Tea will be served on the train and milk for the children. A meal will be provided shortly after your arrival in London.

Identity Cards and Ration Books.

Be sure to take your Identity Cards and all your Ration Books with you. See that the names and addresses of the retailers (including the milkman) with whom you are registered are entered in the Ration Books before you leave.

Go to the Food Office as soon as possible after you get home and take with you your Identity Cards as well as all your Ration Books.

Medical Examination of Children.

The children will be medically examined at Somerset House at 10 a.m. on Monday June 11th 45.

Please make sure that your children attend for this examination.

Yours faithfully,

[illegible signature]

Billeting Officer.

CHAPTER THREE

LIFE AFTER WAR

The war was over, but for us there was another battle to fight. After returning from evacuation, my parents set about pursuing my continuing education. State schools treated any request for entry as if I had the plague. My parents were trying their best to secure a "normal" life for me, but I was starting to realise that my splinted arm was branding me as something of a freak of nature. I decided to fight back!

Despite only being paralysed in one arm, it was said that I could not go to the local school, which was just five minutes away. There was no special school locally, so the Education Authority of the time was not very interested in finding me a place. My parents wrote countless letters to the authorities, but months passed without action. I was almost eight by this time; I had had only three months in infant school before being excluded because of my splinted arm being stuck in the air and about eight months at the special school in Yorkshire. I was desperate to attend school and learn to read books.

I remember an interview with the local Education Officer; I noticed particularly his white hair, his horn-rimmed spectacles - and his stupidity. He asked me lots of silly questions, so I decided to be very brief in my answers in the hope that this would stop him asking more. I know I confused a two shilling piece with half a crown and it was obvious he then thought me as stupid as he was. The outcome was that I was to be allowed to attend school in the London area of Plumstead. The school was mostly a bombed-out shell where two classes of children were taught; one class was mentally handicapped and the other physically so.

My mother took me on a long bus ride each school day to a place called Abbey Wood, where I was put on a school bus. I liked that - at least I had some company of my own age and we used to sing hymns, one of which I particularly remember:

Jesus bids us shine with a pure clear light,
Like a little candle shining in the night,
He looks down from heaven to see us shine,
You in your small corner and me in mine.

I have been an atheist for many years, but I've never forgotten those lovely lines and I have determinedly been passionately trying to shine ever since, perhaps sometimes rather wastefully.

The school in Plumstead was not a great success. I was frightened by some of the mentally ill pupils. Nobody seemed to take the trouble to explain why those unfortunate children behaved the way they did. Winter came and there was heavy snow. One day we were sent home early, but the school bus only went as far as Abbey Wood, where I was left standing outside a pub at 2 pm. I had to wait there until 4 pm, when my mother came to take me the rest of the way home. She was furious that I had been left standing alone for so long in such awful weather and decided that I should not go back to that school. I so envied the children in our road, who could all go to the local schools together, chattering as they walked. As an only child, I had only my Mum to talk to and play with on school days.

So at eight years old, the battle for my education resumed. My parents decided that the only way was to send me to a private school. They contacted the local convent. They weren't particularly keen to have me - not being a catholic - but suggested a school one-and-a-half miles from my home. It was run by two sisters in a semi-detached house in Erith Road, Barnhurst, Kent. Miss Jones and her sister, whom we called Miss Edith, were rather frightening. Miss Jones had white hair cut into a short bob; she was the older of the two and crippled with arthritis. She always seemed to wear pinky-coloured blouses and longish skirts with shoes that had a buttoned strap. She seemed very tall, but then I suppose I was very small.

Miss Edith was mousy, wore similar clothes, clicked her false teeth and was strict but less fair than her sister. Discipline and good manners were paramount. The three R's were thoroughly taught and the whole foundation of my education was laid in this school during my four years there from aged 8 to 12 years. It was here that I learned to read and write. I do not remember being treated any differently from my fellow pupils, although my arm was still in a splint for my first three years there. I never felt any different from the able-bodied children. In all, there were about 30 pupils in two classes at this school.

Our classrooms were the back room downstairs and the front room upstairs. The front room downstairs was the Misses Jones' sitting room and office. We only entered this one if we had committed a serious misdemeanour, which had to be discussed in private. We were only allowed into the kitchen when we had reached a more senior level, to collect warm milk for the students, for which our parents paid 3d per week. The garden was used in the summer for team games. I was once summoned to the front sitting room/office for the terrible crime of telling a lie. I had desperately wanted my parents to have another child, but alas they had opted not to because of the war and my polio. So I decided to invent a baby brother! On the way to school, I told a man in the bus queue that my mother had a new baby. He seemed to show an interest, so I decided to maintain the fiction, so much so that I think I came to believe it!

Friday was the day when we were expected to thank God in our morning assembly for something – so I thanked Him for my baby brother! It caused quite a stir and everyone asked lots of questions about him, but after several weeks I got fed up with this and told them that the baby had gone to Heaven. Everyone was very sympathetic, which just made it even worse. Things quietened down and I hoped it had all been forgotten, but then my mother went to pay my school fees and Miss Jones sympathised over the loss of the baby! The dreadful truth was out - that I had lied and, worse still, had invented the poor baby's death. I was sent to face Miss Jones in that front room.

She was oh so tall and oh so angry! I felt very frightened when she asked me why I lied. I tried to say that everyone misunderstood me, but of course I did not fool her. I can't remember my punishment - only my agonising shame, especially when later that day I had to face my parents, who could not understand why I had done it. After that my longings were kept to myself, but I pledged that if I ever married I would not have just one lonely child, as I had been. To this day, I feel guilty that my polio was the only reason my parents did not have another child.

When I was 12, the Misses Jones retired from school teaching and sold the house. This was a sad blow to my family; it meant another go at getting me into a state school, with three more years of formal education to complete before I became 15 (the school leaving age then) in 1952. Another battle started to get me into the local secondary school. As I no longer wore a splint on my arm this should not have been a problem. All my treatment had been stopped and the hospital said there was nothing else that could be done for me. I suppose I had now realised that my paralysis was for life.

It was only the intervention of Margaret Roberts, who later became Britain's first woman Prime Minister, Mrs Thatcher, that actually got me back to school when she wrote the County Council..

My mother, meanwhile, never lacked tenacity and decided it was not yet time to give up the struggle to improve my distorted right arm. She discovered a Mr Waters, an ex-boxer turned masseur; he was a dark handsome and very muscular man in his late 30s/early 40s. He thought he could help me, but the treatment was very costly, about £21 for 28 treatments, which was a considerable sum then. My mother said she would find the money somehow. She learned to crochet - fortunately much in fashion at the time - and sat long hours day and night making doilies, dressing table sets, string bags and all kinds of decorations, selling when and where she could.

Mr Waters regularly massaged my arm and taught me to do as many exercises as possible; I had little dumbbells with lead weights on the end that I had to try to push into the air. I enjoyed the visits and the pleasure it gave my parents when I realised any small aims, but in truth I think the improvements were mostly imaginary. I did learn a few tricks of using muscles that did work to make more movements normally done in other ways, but it wasn't until many years later that I discovered how to use these tricks to fool myself into thinking I could make my arm work better.

I can't remember for how long Mr Waters visited my home. Eventually, the visits ended, but my parents did not give up. They heard of a healer in Cornwall and somehow the money was saved to take me there with other children. I was fascinated by Cornwall, which seemed like a foreign country to me. We had cake for breakfast – very odd! - But everyone was extremely kind and the whitewashed cottage where we stayed was very homely and comfortable.

My father joined me in seeing the healer; his ankylosing spondylitis had left him permanently bent over with a severe stoop. The healer was a little balding man, in a small room with a huge padded sofa on which he stood. He asked my father to stand in front of him with his back towards the healer. Then he put his arms under those of my father and suddenly yanked him up from the floor. My father went dead white and looked dreadful. I didn't want him to hurt my Dad and desperately hoped he would not do it again because I thought I would cry if he did. Then he turned to me, he felt my back and shoulders and said I had a dislocated spine near my neck. He pulled and pushed me and then suddenly wound my arm in a great circle and then it was over. Neither my father nor I had any long term improvement from this treatment.

One of my other Cornish memories was very frightening. We were among a number of people who had made the trip west for the same purpose as my family and it was decided to visit the beach at Padstow. We were all greatly enjoying ourselves and were not watching the incoming tide, which is very fast there. Suddenly someone noticed that we had been cut off. The beach was backed with steep rocks forming a bay and the water was lapping over the rocks on both sides leaving only the sandy expanse we were sitting on. The only way to get away was up the rocks. But some of those with us were suffering the effects of polio in their legs and climbing for them was very hard. Somehow we managed to scramble up the cliff, but our way then lay along a footpath which involved us all in a very long walk through fields where cattle were grazing - much to my mother's consternation.

She was convinced they were all bulls just waiting to attack us! We eventually returned to our lodgings very tired but none the worse for our experiences.

I also vividly remember seeing a strange fruit in a shop window. My parents said it was a pomegranate; they bought one and took it home for me to eat. My father just cut it in half and laid it before me. I was most curious but thought I ought to remove the seeds before beginning to eat it. I put them all in a pile on the side of the plate, then promptly burst into tears as there was nothing left for me to eat. My parents were very amused and explained that you had to eat the seeds, which I thought was most peculiar.

We returned from Cornwall no worse, maybe a little better, for our experiences, but as yet my parents were still not ready to give up the struggle to improve my wasted arm. They heard about a faith healer in Bromley, Kent, and from then on for many months we travelled by bus on an awkward journey every Saturday to this man's home, where we all sat around a central plinth on which the patient lay. The healer laid his hands on the effected part while several assistants stood around with outstretched hands. Music played constantly on a record player and I can never hear the sound of 'The Dream of Olwen' or 'Oh Mein Papa' without thinking of all those boring Saturday afternoons when my parents were doing their very best to improve my lot.

I suppose even they eventually had to accept that no amount of love or money could restore the wasted muscles of my right arm, and anyway my life did not seem particularly difficult. I wasn't very good at games, but I didn't particularly enjoy them so it mattered very little. I learned to sew, knit and cook things that were a joy to me. I can no longer knit because of pain in my 'good' shoulder. My sewing these days tends to be limited to repairs, maintenance and fancy dress costumes for my granddaughters, but cooking is still great fun to me and thoroughly enjoyable, as is eating. My figure proves that!

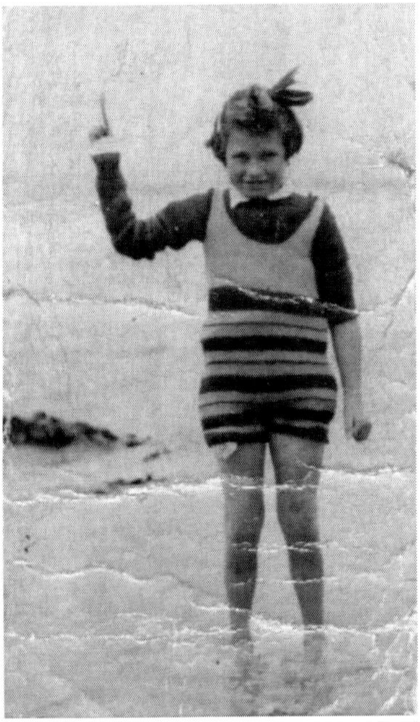

Left - Margate shortly before I broke my arm trying to jump over a deck chair.

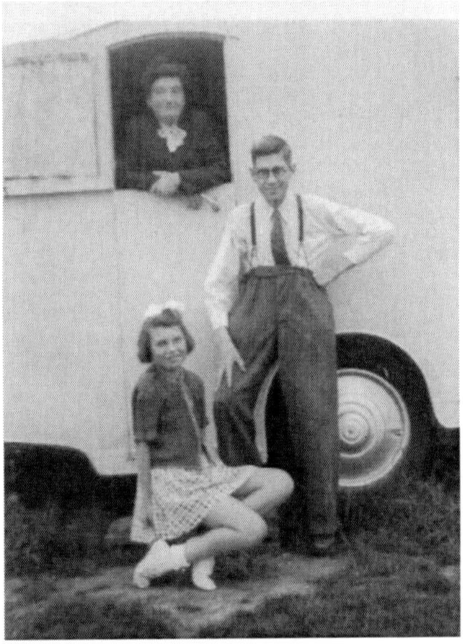

Right – aged 10 on our first holiday as a family after the war. My splint had been removed for the photo.

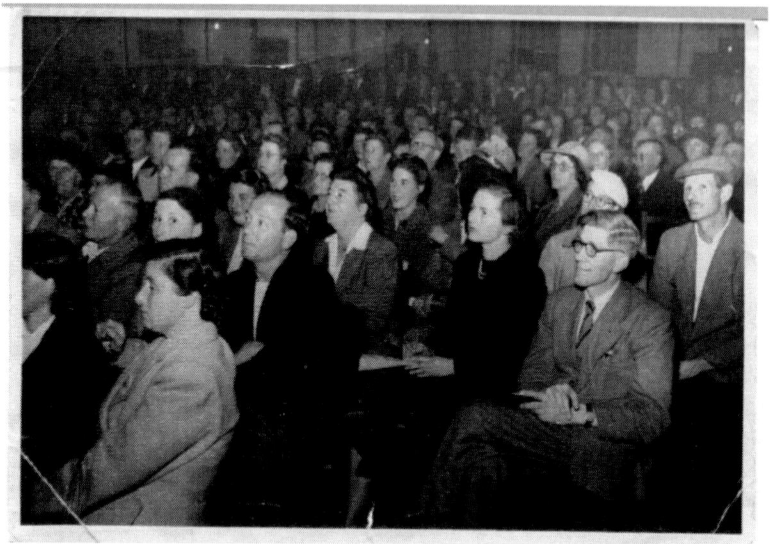

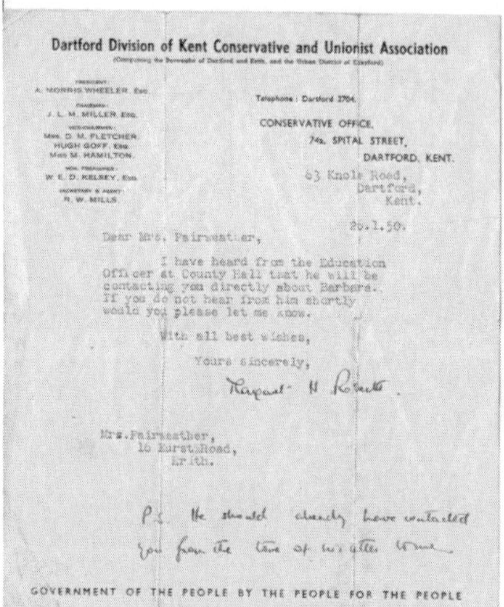

Dartford Division of Kent Conservative and Unionist Association

A. MORRIS WHEELER, Esq.
J. L. M. MILLER, Esq.
Mrs. D. M. FLETCHER
HUGH GOFF, Esq.
Miss M. HAMILTON
W. E. D. KELSEY, Esq.
R. W. MILLS

Telephone: Dartford 2704.

CONSERVATIVE OFFICE,
74a, SPITAL STREET,
DARTFORD, KENT.

63 Knole Road,
Dartford,
Kent.

20.1.50.

Dear Mrs. Fairweather,

I have heard from the Education Officer at County Hall that he will be contacting you directly about Barbara. If you do not hear from him shortly would you please let me know.

With all best wishes,

Yours sincerely,

Margaret H Roberts.

Mrs. Fairweather,
16 Hurst Road,
Erith.

P.S. He should already have contacted you from the time of [illegible]

GOVERNMENT OF THE PEOPLE BY THE PEOPLE FOR THE PEOPLE

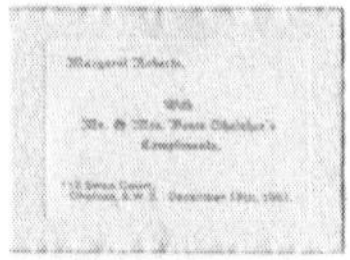

Above photo: Miss Roberts with my parents whilst electioneering in 1950.

Left: Letter to my Mother.

Above: Card sent to my parents with wedding cake when she married & became Mrs Thatcher, the first woman Prime Minister of Britain.

ADMINISTRATION OF THE COUNTY OF KENT

Miss D. E. HARVIE, B. Sc.
Children's Officer.
Telephone:
Maidstone 4395.
Extn. 536
Your Ref.:

Please quote my reference: DEH/MFD

County Hall,
Maidstone.

7th January, 1950

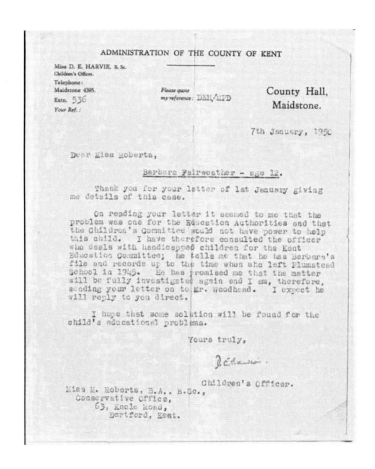

Dear Miss Roberts,

Barbara Fairweather - age 12.

Thank you for your letter of 1st January giving me details of this case.

On reading your letter it seemed to me that the problem was one for the Education Authorities and that the Children's Committee would not have power to help this child. I have therefore consulted the officer who deals with handicapped children for the Kent Education Committee; he tells me that he has Barbara's file and records up to the time when she left Plumstead School in 1945. He has promised me that the matter will be fully investigated again and I am, therefore, sending your letter on to Mr. Woodhead. I expect he will reply to you direct.

I hope that some solution will be found for the child's educational problems.

Yours truly,

D.E.Harvie.

Children's Officer.

Miss M. Roberts, B.A., B.Sc.,
Conservative Office,
63, Knole Road,
Dartford, Kent.

Reply to Margaret Roberts Letter.

CHAPTER FOUR

EARLY TEENAGE YEARS

After I left the private school at 12 years and was finally accepted at the local Secondary School – only to be faced with a new challenge of a very different kind. My polio arm was no longer splinted, so it posed no "threat" to the other children. However, the fact that I had attended a private school, and had been well taught in grammar and speech, meant that I did not fit in too well in my new educational environment. I had been trained to work hard and to be very obedient. So I was considered 'different', too much of a 'goody, goody' child and snooty for having been educated privately.

This was a tough working class area, times were hard for most people, and an only child from my background was definitely considered odd. I don't think my classmates meant to be cruel, but like anyone who does not fit into the group image I was somewhat ostracised. I was lonely there and never formed any close friendships as I had done at my previous school. Consequently, I learned to stand on my own two feet and aim for the top. Had I been in my peers' shoes, I would no doubt have behaved as they did. Of course, an obedient, hardworking student was very popular with the teachers. My reports were excellent and I was soon placed in the top stream, even becoming a prefect. My fellow pupils finally voted for me to become their House Captain, which made me very proud. So I suppose at the end of my school life I gained some respect, if not the love, of my peers.

When I was about 13, the puppy fat began to appear and I could not hide my developing bust, so I asked Mum for a bra. Money for new was not readily available, so she found one of her older, flesh-pink, stiffly-boned numbers which I proudly wore to school the next day - promptly informing my friends of my new adult status symbol. After lunch many better-endowed pupils, plus a few with mere bumps, returned to class wearing an assortment of brassieres that would now be regarded as museum pieces!

Another "adult" milestone now was my first period, which I mention to record the only sanitary protection available to poor women at this time. Pads were made from a double square of material about 10 inches (25cm) square, cut from the better parts of worn-out white sheets. A loop of tape about one inch long was sewn at diagonal corners. The opposite corners were folded across each other to form the pad, which was then held in place by a piece of tape that went around the waist, through the loops at the back and front of the pad, and tied in a bow. The whole thing was bulky and inefficient and had to be wrapped in newspaper and taken home for washing when soiled. (Hence the need to carry large hand or shopping bags. Plastic bags were not available at this time.) Every home had an enamel bucket with a lid; this was filled with cold water and generally stood in the woman's bedroom. Soiled pads were placed in the bucket to soak before being boiled in the copper. My grandmother, who had four daughters, used to hang the washed cloths on a line beneath the mantelshelf and tell her sons they were dusters. The mantelshelf had a velour cloth around it, presumably to hide the offending articles.

At 14, I was miserable; I was sure no-one loved me. I was too old to play with my younger cousins, but too young in the eyes of the family to wear make-up, high heels, nylon stockings, low-necked dresses, or to stay out after 8 pm unless with parents. My father expected my clothes to cover everything between neck and knees. I hated most of all the navy blue bloomer type knickers that were school uniform. In the school play, I was given the part of a Holy Bonze (a Japanese or Chinese priest). My costume was a white bed sheet held together with pins topped with a black felt hat cut from the crown of an old school hat. The rehearsals went well, with no speeches to learn, as it was all in mime, and the acting had to convey the scene to the audience.

This was my big chance! It was opening night before the Mayor, the Bishop of Rochester and assembled parents and friends. I stood in the wings, with the excitement and nerves mounting. I was determined to put everything into my shuffle across that stage and my reverent bow. Alas, for me, it was definitely NOT "all right on the night!" The curtains opened, I shuffled, I bowed, I stepped forward centre stage – only to tread on my flowing robe, sending the bed-sheet sliding to the floor! Revealed was a 14-year-old dumpling in a white vest and navy blue bloomers with one thin short arm and one fat chubby one! I heard the gasp and slight titter run around the audience as I rushed from the stage in acute embarrassment. For some reason, I always got comedy roles after that.

It was about this time that I had my first perm, which was done by a local hairdresser who had converted a bedroom into a salon at her home. She had a big machine for perming hair electrically. I remember a stand with a large circle at the top from which hung the roller covers that were placed over the curlers. The curlers had to be wound ringlet-fashion with the perming lotion on them; the covers were then pushed over them and the machine turned on to heat the perming lotion. The covers were very heavy and I remember thinking my neck would break under the weight. If left too long, the hair would just burn away, so it could be a very dangerous affair. Generally, though, the result was a very dry frizzy head of hair. I was not too keen on a repeat performance!

My last year at secondary school was crowned with a part in the play 'Women at War,' set in the time of Cromwell. I was an 80-year-old rebel who refused to dress with the simplicity required of Cromwellian women. I appeared in a voluminous pink and black crinoline, high hat with numerous feathers, a knobbly walking stick in my good hand and a muff to hide the short arm. My generous flesh was held by a stomacher - a front-piece of 16th-17th Century dress covering breast and pit of stomach, ending in a point over the skirt. At a high point in the drama I had to rise from my chair complaining that I was just a bag of bones. I rose, knocking over the heavy Jacobean side table, glasses and biscuits with a resounding crash! The local paper said I played my part on a clowning level! That concluded my early acting career!

When I was 14, my father was struck down with a recurrence of his stomach ulcer problems which, combined with his ankylosing spondylitis, almost killed him. This was a terrible time for the family, as he lay curled up in agony day after day for months on end. His weight dropped below nine stone and money worries worsened as his salary was cut to half pay.

During this time I had bought home a letter from my school saying they were running a trip to Paris. This was an 'out of this world' experience in the post-war Britain of 1952, a very exciting prospect for a working class child whose experience of anywhere beyond these shores was limited to geography books. I gave no thought to how my parents might find the £28 required to pay for the trip plus pocket money. I rushed home, wreathed in smiles, to tell them. Then reality struck when my father said I could not go; the money was not there because he was so ill and could not work. My disappointment must have been obvious, but my mother's indomitable spirit triumphed again. She was determined I should go; she found work in a shoe shop, crocheted and sewed as well as looking after my ailing father. Somehow she got together enough money to pay for that trip.

Paris . . . WHAT an experience! The train we took from Calais had only hard wooden benches and seemed very dirty and smelly. Every child brought sandwiches with them to eat on the way. When we reached the great city, I remember the sooty blackness of all the buildings, which quite shocked me. I hated the strong smell of garlic on the breath of those people travelling in the Metro underground and I was confused by the babble of voices in a language I didn't understand.

Our hotel was a tall narrow building squashed between others in a narrow back street. It was very dark inside, the predominant colours being brown, black and mustard. Dingy net curtains covered the French windows in our bedroom. Mattresses were slung over the balcony rails of windows on the opposite side of the street. It was all quite a shock to me, coming from a home where everything was clean, bright and polished.

Breakfast was not what I was used to at home, either, with slices of rather dry baguette and a little jam with strong coffee, which I hated. Breakfast at home came with tea, or if I had coffee Mum made it with half a teaspoon of Nescafe topped up with hot milk. French food did not impress my English palette that was used to the simple, plain wartime diet.

I enjoyed visiting the palace at Versailles as I was always keen on learning history and everything related. I remember Les Invalides because I tripped on a marble step, falling on my face and splitting my lip. The Eiffel Tower was exciting, as was the freedom from parental control! My secret supply of lipstick and eye shadow enabled me to believe I was irresistible to the opposite sex. I hoped I also looked at least 17 - but the split lip ruined the image! I don't think the puppy fat did much for me, either!

As an all-female group, we giggled a lot in the hotel, much to the chagrin of an elderly French resident. He came out of his room wearing long yellowing underpants and vest, both very baggy. He angrily let forth a stream of abuse in language we did not comprehend. This further increased our giggles until our horrified teacher appeared to chastise us and apologise to the old gentleman. Another sight that shocked me was a woman dressed all in black fishing in the dustbins for thrown-away food. I saw her retrieve a long bread stick from the hotel bin and hurry off with it.

We were not allowed to drink wine or go out in the evenings except once when our teachers took us for a walk along the Champs Elysées to see the lights and stop at a cafe. I thought it was very magical, although we were kept well under control. French boys were considered by our teachers to be most unsuitable and on no account were we to go near them. I was fascinated by the Mona Lisa painting and the Venus de Milo statue in the Louvre museum. For the return journey, each child received two slices of dry, unbuttered bread and a hard-boiled egg for the train journey to Dover.

I had become interested in art and decided when I left school at 15 that I would like to go to art school. I passed an entrance exam to attend Bromley College of Art, which greatly pleased my parents. I began there after Christmas, 1952. This was the beginning of my slightly 'Bohemian' period, although parental control prevented me from dressing exactly as I wished. I must have looked a very strange sight in my long dangling earrings and home-made 'jelly bag' hats which were all the rage worn with thick polo neck sweaters – a ghastly ensemble topped off with a college scarf of which I was extremely proud!

Generally, I enjoyed the freer way of life at college and made friends more easily. I also enjoyed the mixed company. Young men were fascinating, but somewhat frightening - my last school had been all girls. I don't think I was a particularly appealing teenager because of my weight and lack of dress sense. I was certain no-one would find me attractive because the polio had so distorted my right arm and left it about five inches shorter than my left arm. I decided I would never marry and because of this I would throw myself into college work and evening school.

At college I particularly remember two boys who were training to become milliners. One was the great Graham Smith, who later made hats for the very rich and famous, including the late Princess of Wales; the other was nicknamed 'Chunky.' Graham was thin and willowy, Chunky square and sturdy, but both were cheery chaps with a great sense of humour. They amused me no end, especially when their creations often ended up on their own heads! The girls were great fun, too, and none of us took life too seriously. We had a common room in an attic at the top of an old house used by the college in Tweedy Road, Bromley. Up there we had old sofas and chairs where we sat smoking Turkish cigarettes and creating a blue haze in the closed attic room. We thought ourselves very grown-up and trendy!

About the time I started college, sweets were de-rationed. It was so exciting to buy a whole bar of chocolate or a packet of Spangles fruit sweets. It seemed so greedy not to share, so I ate mine in secret until I got over the novelty. Occasionally we bunked off college and went to the local Pullman cinema, which was considered very daring. We saw blockbusters like the

American 'Quo Vadis' and many of the films made in the great British studios at Shepperton and Elstree.

I did my best at college, but I soon realised that I was not the most creative or accomplished student; my talents probably lay elsewhere. My parents would not hear of me changing courses, though, so I would have to stick it out for some time to come.

For almost three years, I enjoyed and sometimes endured college life. I regularly swapped my ham or cheese sandwiches for a girl friend's constant supply of peanut butter sandwiches. Heather and I used to sit on the radiators in the locker room eating our lunch and gossiping. We are grey-haired matrons now, but we chat about those days and still enjoy a good gossip. In the evenings, we made cocoa in milk bottles, using our paintbrushes to stir the revolting mixture.

Outside college, I went to evening classes three nights a week at a local grammar school, studying English language, English literature and history. I can still quote examples of alliteration from 'The Ancient Mariner' from those days, a very useful talent in later life! My two-hour journey enabled me to do all my homework before it went out of my head. By the time I got the bus and train home, it was nearly 11 pm and I fell into bed exhausted.

One night a week I was an ardent 'Young Conservative,' going to the local club in Belvedere. I played table tennis there and served on the committee, but I remember little about our political activities - more about the young men I met there. At weekends I got up later as I loved to read in bed. It was also the place where I dreamt about my future. I don't think my dreams ever included a long marriage, children and grandchildren. I saw a flat in London, a career and travel; I did not bargain for Rod – but that's another chapter!

Weekends were fun, with visits to record shops with a boy from college, when we could squeeze into a little record booth to listen to traditional jazz records which we sometimes bought. Frequently I visited the cinema, where the big film always seemed to be accompanied by a western. It never seemed to matter that you went in part way through the film; you just sat there until the film came round again and then watched the beginning until you caught up with it. Nearly everyone smoked, so you watched the film through a cloud and was conscious of all the coughing only when it became quietly tense during a romantic or frightening scene. Occasionally there would be a wit in the audience who would make a comment, which made everyone laugh. Generally, the girls enjoyed the romance and the boys the westerns. I don't ever remember anyone being aggressive, perhaps because we mostly drank in coffee bars and played the latest hits on the jukebox. There were lots of 'Teddy Boys' and their girls, but they seemed to be more concerned for their dress and DA (Duck's Arse) haircuts than causing fights. I thought their great crepe soled shoes and drainpipe trainers very ugly. I swam with my girlfriends often, wrote lots of letters to family and friends because few of them were on the telephone, and read a great many books. Mum and Dad had a gramophone on which I played my records. I listened to plays on the radio and learnt to make my own clothes.

My father had heard of The Infantile Paralysis Fellowship (now The BPF), a national organisation for the welfare and support of polio victims who also benefited from local group social meetings. My father was very active in helping the fellowship in my teenage years and became its chairman. I, too, was a busy committee member, organising outings, fund-raising and social events. I thoroughly enjoyed organising, as I still do, and the outings were great fun. The younger members always tried to congregate at the back of the coach, where we could sing all sorts of saucy songs and puff a few forbidden cigarettes when Mum and Dad weren't looking. We had no idea that smoking could kill, but I suspect we would not have worried anyway because we regarded old age (i.e. anyone over 25) as being far, far away and not relative to us! We wanted to look older and more sophisticated, but we did not want to think like 'old' people.

My new sophisticated image was very evident on one coach outing when I wore a blue straw beret-shaped hat with a neat little veil over the forehead and eyes. On the back seat, my friend and I had secretly acquired some of those forbidden cigarettes. I lit a match, but quite forget the little veil - which immediately flared as I touched the cigarette, setting the hat on fire. I screamed and a friend grabbed the hat from my head, quickly smothering the smouldering straw. I suffered nothing worse than a singed fringe and scorched eyebrows, but the attention of the full coach load of people was drawn to me and I was terrified of the wrath of my parents at the front. They said very little, though, and years later I realised the event had caused much mirth among my fellow travellers. Among them, though, was a St John Ambulance first aider, who warned us not to mix hats and smoking again!

On seaside outings, we sang all sorts of songs - some saucy, some old favourites, some where the coach was divided into groups for different parts of the singing. We did not have to worry about drinking and driving, so after a pub stop on the way back the adult members of the party were more relaxed. The singing became livelier and less inhibited; a few rugby songs began to creep into our repertoire!

When we disembarked from the coach, out would come all the wheelchairs, crutches and walking sticks. There were very few aids for the disabled then, so the able-bodied members lifted and heaved everyone out of the coach amid a lot of banter and joking. Lunch was usually arranged and involved lots more struggling to get all the disabled to their seats at long tables, but it was all very good-humoured.

I never saw any political correctness or demonstrating against 'the system.' We had suffered misfortune, yes, but we never saw ourselves as victims. We just tried to be as normal as possible and accepted our frustration as our own problem. Self-help groups for social and welfare purposes were formed with families and a few sympathetic friends, but nothing like today's efforts. It is good to know that people are more aware today, but trust, love of life, friendship and most of all a sense of fun seem less evident. Laughter relieves pain more than aggression.

CHAPTER FIVE

ROMANCE

I wonder what today's archetypal "modern," street-wise, sexually active youngster would make of the mid-teen me?! Apart from the very basic facts of life, I had little knowledge of sex or the male physique. The attractions I felt for the opposite sex had more to do with natural development than actual experience. With no siblings and a quiet, very reserved and non-sporty father, my only role models came from magazines or the highly romantic fictional heroes of films.

When my parents took me, at 16, to a Navy Day at Chatham Dockyard, the sight of all those young, handsome, uniformed sailors was a great thrill to me. We toured submarines, destroyers and battleships, which was very exciting. On one ship, I purposely lost my watchful parents and began talking to a handsome young sailor who asked my name. Alas, I was mortified when, clearly regarding me as a child, he then put out a call on the ship's tannoy for my parents to collect me!

The streets in the years after the war remained full of young men in service uniforms; we still had National Service and most were conscripted for two years. I always preferred men in uniform, and particularly sailors, with their navy blue bell-bottomed trousers, big white collars and jaunty caps. My father's friend had a son of similar age to me; he went straight into boy service in the Navy when he left school. I really liked him, but it was another case of unrequited love. This good-looking lad with dark curly hair was a painfully shy 'Adonis' who never gave me the slightest encouragement. Many years later (when I was a grandmother), I was just leaving work and was stopped by a chubby bald-headed man who said, 'Excuse me, aren't you Barbara Fairweather?'

'Yes, I was,' I replied, 'but I'm afraid I don't know you.'

'I'm Johnny. Remember - our dads were mates. I went into the navy after school.'

I hoped he was not hurt that I did not recognise him, especially when he said I had not changed much. That made me realise that my puppy fat had grown old with me and was now called middle-aged spread! We chatted for a while and then he told me he was going to work in Saudi Arabia within a few days. We laughed a lot about the past, particularly when I told him how I had thought myself madly in love with him as a teenager! I never saw him again.

My first romantic kiss was with a college mate who I will just call D. He had for some time accompanied me to silent film shows after our art classes and we seemed to get along well so when my Mum let me have a 16th Birthday party at home I invited D. After the party I walked to the bus stop with him in the pouring rain, where he kissed me as we stood under an archway. It was lovely (well, I thought it was) and I walked back home on cloud nine but I soon fell off it with quite a bump! Whether it was the ride home or me I have no idea! He, on the other hand, must have thought it very uncomfortable sitting in his very wet clothes on the long ride home which must have cooled his ardour somewhat! It certainly had cooled by the time I met him again. We went our separate ways after that and I believe he became a very successful artist in America.

As for my next romantic date, it was ruined by my mother insisting that I wore a hideous hat decorated across the front with beads. I knew it would be a disaster; I wished I had stuck to my original plan which was to throw it in the river and tell Mum it had blown away in the wind. My courage failed me and, as I expected, the date was not repeated. I always seemed to have a problem with hats!

Then, while I was away on holiday with my mother, I received a postcard from a friend, Maureen, telling me that a new chap had joined the British Polio Fellowship club to which we both belonged. She seemed impressed and said although he had a paralysed leg he was a very active and energetic 20-year-old. This man was to change the rest of my life! Maureen introduced me to Rodney on return from my holiday and the three of us played darts together. The club met every Thursday evening and often we joined in the group activities, although I had no special interest in him then. I think my friend might have done, but sadly for her it did not work out.

Six months after our first meeting, the club ran a trip to a party for polio victims in London. It was early December, 1954. I was just 17 and looking forward to the annual event where we met people from all over the country. Vera Lynn frequently came with stars from the theatre, so we really enjoyed ourselves. On the return coach trip, Rod asked me to sit with him. We hung our paper hats on the ashtrays behind the seats in front of us and he nervously pinged the elastic on mine for a while before asking me to go to the cinema with him one evening. As small beginnings go, it was indeed small – not the stuff of romantic novels, and not love at first sight or seeing stars or hearing bells – but it heralded the start of our long relationship.

I happily went to an ice show with Rod a few days later. Ice shows in London then were very spectacular with what seemed like a cast of hundreds in very colourful costumes. Because of the absence of TV, such shows always had a great impact on us. I loved watching the figures gliding so elegantly across the wide expanse of ice and the funny men who fell over and seemed to get it all wrong.

My diary for the end of 1954 records my love for Rod, but I don't think he impressed my parents too much because of an incident when we were left alone for the first time one evening in their home, early in the New Year. The light bulb in the centre of the living room went pop and I asked Rod if he could replace it. He climbed onto the table, reached up to grasp the flex holding the fitting - and succeeded in bringing the whole thing crashing down! The flex had ripped away from the ceiling rose. He was very worried about what my father would say! On Dad's return, I explained what had happened and he advised: 'There is a switch on the wall if you want to sit in the dark!'

We enjoyed many cinema outings; there were two cinemas in Dartford then, plus a small theatre. There are no cinemas now and the old theatre is a night club and restaurant. All the young men seemed to carry long raincoats, but I suppose in the days when very few had cars the long raincoat was the next best thing. It was used for sitting on in fields, for cuddling up in dark alleyways and for knee and thigh touching in the cinemas! All very innocent by today's standards, but very illicit in the 1950s!

Parents rarely mentioned sex to their children, but it was often a topic with close friends that was more talked about than actually achieved and very exciting to discover slowly. It was not thrust upon us in advertising or in films. The moral high ground always seemed to triumph in the films! Perhaps it was unrealistic and innocence was probably the downfall of many a girl.

Rod had a very jolly group of friends and during our courtship we joined them hiking in the local countryside and drinking in a club that belonging to Rod's employers. We would also visit each other's family homes. There were frequent parties, social evenings, picnics and an occasional trip to a pub. We had little money, but always plenty to do.

I recall one hike when the fashion for tapered trousers had arrived. I was very proud of mine; they were black and white check, topped off with a grey checked swagger jacket. We walked up hill and down dale, over fields and across stiles - but one of these was my downfall. As I cocked my leg over the top bar of the stile, my ample rear stretched the fabric of my trousers to breaking point. RIP! They were split from waistbands to crotch, revealing my knickers to the merry party following me! Hoots of laughter echoed through the woodland, much to my embarrassment! To my rescue came one of the girls in the group who always had emergency supplies. To my relief, these included needle and cotton. She was nicknamed 'Miss Efficiency' after that. The only trouble was she had firmly sewn my knickers to my trousers!

I was still at college when I met Rod in 1954 but left in May 1955 to start work. Later that same year in August, Rod was 21 and his parents threw a party for him. He amazed me with his ability to join in everything and to be the life and soul of the party with total disregard for his polio leg - despite his pronounced limp, with his very thin right leg; he certainly did not seem to notice it. I admired him because the handicap made little difference to him and his friends, although I was always conscious of my own paralysed arm, I always hid in corners at dances. In this respect, he was the exact opposite of me.

Rod was a trainee scientific glassblower with the pharmaceutical firm Burroughs Wellcome & Co. Ltd. Our courting was normally on Wednesday evenings, Saturday and Sundays. Much of the summer was spent walking around the fields and woods that Rod had enjoyed all his life. The country life was very new to me and sometimes far less idyllic than I had imagined. He lived in Wilmington, Dartford, which was still very much a village then. His home was a little terraced cottage two doors from The Plough pub. His father was a farm labourer; his home had originally been one in a row of tied cottages belonging to the Carpenter's Farm where he worked. The rooms were quite small, the toilet was in the yard, and there was no bathroom or bath. In the back yard stood a large mangle used for wringing out the washing. Next to the outside loo was a coal cupboard, which also doubled as a place to hang garden implements. Rod bathed once a week in the clubhouse at his work; the rest of the time, the family washed at the kitchen sink.

My first visit to his home was a peep into a lifestyle essentially new to me. His parents and brother were all very down to earth - very blunt talkers, and not bothered by a little mud in the house. They were simple, happy country folk. Food was basic, usually fresh and very hearty. Much fat was consumed. Roasts were deep in lard and pastry was thick. Puddings full of suet were boiled in tea cloths. Soup, fortified with pearl barley and lentils, was so thick you could stand a spoon up in it. Milk was the gold top variety, with extra cream. There were plenty of fresh vegetables and seasonal fruit. Bread was cut into big doorsteps, thickly spread with real butter. Tea was the main drink, but Camp (liquid essence) coffee was the mid-morning drink when at home, made entirely with hot milk.

On one of my early visits to the cottage I came across raw beetroot, which I did not recognise as it was uncooked. When told what it was, I greatly amused the family by saying I had 'never seen live beetroot before!' After that, the family always referred to uncooked beetroot as being 'live'.

I loved going out with Rod and his parents in his father's tiny Austin 7 car for a picnic. They took a little tin kettle and a methylated spirit stove to boil water for tea. We sat in the fields eating sandwiches, cake and fruit on idyllic summer days. This was a phase of my life that proved all too short – as you will see later.

Our relationship had now deepened and Rod and I were viewed as a pair (or an 'item,' as the modern term has it) by family and friends. In those days, if you were taken to visit relations by a boyfriend you were considered to be in a steady relationship.

I had left college in 1955 to start work in 1956; one of our walks in the woods took us to a pig farm. I loved pigs and collected those ornaments, that is, not live ones! After we watched the animals for a while, we sat on the grass nearby and that is where Rod proposed. Such a romantic place to be asked for one's hand in marriage! All the same, I said yes. We told our parents, adding that we hoped to get engaged on my 19th birthday in November, when we would have saved enough to buy a ring for each other. Our parents did not seem particularly overjoyed. Mine thought me too young and, as I had not been in work for very long they considered marriage was not sensible for some time to come. Rod's mother was not pleased that he was thinking of marrying a girl with a paralysed arm because, as he was disabled, she considered he would not be best cared for by someone else with a disability. They did eventually accept the idea in principle, but my father said he would not give his permission for me to marry until I was 21, which was still the age of consent then.

The engagement plans went ahead and my parents arranged a party at the club where the polio victims met so that they could join in with the family in celebrating the occasion. A week before the party, we collected the engagement rings that had been specially made. I was so excited when I saw my sparkling solitaire gold and platinum ring and Rod's gold signet ring beautifully carved with his initials. Then, during a Saturday night dance at Acacia Hall, we decided to slip out into the grounds to exchange rings secretly, prior to the 'official' ceremony arranged by my parents for the following Thursday. It was a fairly dark night and we made our way to a romantic stone seat hidden amongst the trees. The seat was very cold, but I was so happy and thrilled when Rod placed the ring on my finger. I knew then that I could not take it off and wear it on a chain around my neck, as had been planned until the party.

Alas, that proved a big mistake which ruined our big day because when we phoned my parents to tell them we had got engaged already my father was furious and threatened to cancel the party! I could not understand his attitude and was very upset and walked out of the phone box in floods of tears. However Mum persuaded Dad to allow the party to go ahead and we had a lovely time with all the members of the North West Kent Branch of the British Polio Fellowship.

CHAPTER SIX

STARTING WORK

I left the Art College in the summer of 1955 and began working in the 'Needlewoman,' a shop in Regent Street, London. I like to think I quickly made an impression there – not least when, after just a few days, the manager ended up sitting on my lap! (I promise you there was a very satisfactory, if somewhat bizarre, explanation - as you will shortly see.)

The Needlewoman sold all the materials required for embroidery, which was very much in vogue at the time, particularly amongst the upper classes, the acting profession and MPs' wives. Queen Mary, mother of George VI, had created much interest in needlework tapestry work when she had designed and embroidered a carpet of flowers. (I was told later that she only embroidered the actual flowers, with all the background work being completed by The Royal School of Needlework.) Many women made their own clothes and those of their children, so patterns were a large part of the trade, as were embroidery frames, tapestry patterns and silks, cottons, materials, needles of every shape and size and for all purposes.

The staff were strictly controlled. We were never allowed to address each other by our first names when in the shop; it was always Mr, Mrs, or Miss. Shop assistants wore shapeless long dark green overalls, which did nothing for their appearance or morale. The sleeve of my overall, like all long sleeves, had to be shortened by 5 inches (130mm) for my polio arm and I was a bit worried customers might notice but as most customers saw only what they were buying they rarely noticed. Buyers and managers wore their own clothes; they were almighty creatures who expected to be treated with respect, and were. The manager was Mr Firebrace, a dignified man who wore a dark suit and bowler hat and carried a long rolled umbrella.

On my way to work one morning, Mr Firebrace joined my very crowded train at London Bridge; he did not notice me sitting right next to the door. There was standing room only and as the train suddenly jolted forward he was catapulted forward - right into my lap!

"Good morning, Mr Firebrace" I said politely.

"Oh! Miss Fairweather, I'm so sorry!" he exclaimed. The poor man went beetroot-red with embarrassment and confusion at the indignity of sitting on a lowly shop girl, and in full view of so many people. He hastily tried to free himself from this predicament - rising against the pressing throng of passengers – but in so doing only succeeded in falling against me once more. Finally, he managed to hoist his tall frame back into a standing position. It was no great surprise when he ventured nowhere near my counter for the rest of that day.

The girls ate their sandwiches in a dingy basement room beneath the shop. There was no canteen, but we could make tea. I made a couple of good friends there, one of whom joined me later at my next job. I was happy at The Needlewoman but, due to my mother's determination for me to rise to "better things," I left after only three months. My parents felt that being a shop assistant was not a suitable job for me after the training I had received in College. Unknown to me, my mother went to London to search for something she and my father considered more suitable.

That place was The Ladies Work Society. It had been established by a titled lady expressly for distressed gentlewomen to work or obtain a place where their embroidery or antiques could be sold. There was a very dark workshop behind an antique shop. My mother sang my praises to the owner, who agreed to interview me. This lady was the daughter of a baronet and partner of the titled lady who had owned the business originally but had since died. Miss Thorold was an imposing lady with snow-white fine hair, which constantly escaped her bun; her ample bosom heaved as she drew on her expensive cigarettes with beautifully manicured nails. She agreed to take me on for a trial period as an embroidery designer at the magnificent sum of £3.10s (£3.50) per week. Out of this I paid £1 train fares, £1 to my mother for my keep and had stoppages of approximately 4s 6d (22p) for tax and National Insurance. The remainder paid for my lunches, stockings and clothes.

A pair of stockings cost about one third of what I had left. But I paid 1s 0d (5p) to have my frequent ladders repaired by ladies who used to sit in shop windows with an implement like a very fine crochet hook which picked up the threads of the ladder. We were not allowed to go bare-legged – not even on the warmest summer days. Seamless stockings came into fashion at this time and I was the first employee at the LWS to wear them. They were so good that my employer thought I was not wearing stockings at all and asked the manager to reprimand me. He was quite amused when he was told firmly that I was wearing the latest fashion of seamless hose! At least I did not have to wear an overall, but I was expected to wear 'quiet' clothes. Then, when I wore court shoes and a patterned skirt, my employer wrote to my mother asking her to ensure I wore low-healed rubber-soled shoes and darker, plainer clothes.

My first task was to prepare Miss Thorold's afternoon tea tray with her bone china tea service and for this I was shown her special teapot, which she alone used. Her tea was also kept in a separate tin from that of the staff, which I thought rather odd. I was advised that she never took milk. I duly made the tea. It smelled rather scented, which was strange to me as we only had one sort of tea at home. It did not seem very strong - almost colourless, in fact - so I piled in a few more spoonfuls. Big mistake! I carried the tray into the workroom and a separate one for the staff. Miss Thorold always joined us for afternoon tea. She poured, lit her cigarette, took a sip of her tea - and gasped.

'Who made my tea today?' she asked, frowning.

'I did, Miss Thorold,' I replied nervously, 'but it didn't seem to be very strong.'

'My dear girl,' she informed me, 'this is china tea. How much did you put in the pot?'

'About three or four teaspoons, Miss Thorold.'

'Well, please go and make another pot, using about half a teaspoon this time!'

Her tone of voice was very ladylike. I felt she thought me very ignorant and stupid but probably she was more irritated than angry but she certainly wasn't smiling!

That was the first time I learned there was any tea other than the strong brown stuff that we drank at home!

Ironically, I don't think the job was at all what my mother had believed it to be. Certainly it wasn't glamorous, although I did get to serve a few film stars. The nicest of these was Katherine Hepburn, one of the biggest names of them all and a leading lady in Hollywood for more than 60 years. She treated me very much as a fellow human being. She once gave me a handful of 12 sided threepenny pieces because she said she didn't know what to do with them. I explained they were worth three English pennies each but she said the shape was awkward to handle so she wanted me to have them. Sometimes we were given a tip by a grateful customer but the first time that someone gave me a pound the manager said I must politely refuse any gifts. I did say I wasn't allowed to accept money but Miss Hepburn insisted, so I am afraid I accepted, kept the threepenny pieces and kept quiet about it. Now my awful secret is out!

Most of the time I was closeted in the dreary back workroom with two or three other girls and a young male manager. My job did not involve much designing; it was more a case of taking an existing design, tracing it onto canvas and then painting the design in oils. We did a lot of restoration work on needlework tapestries and old embroidered hangings from big country houses. I once spent nine months 'tramming' the linen of a Jacobean hanging from Longleat. This was a process of laying down silk threads over the rotting linen background and catching them down with tiny stitches.

Sometimes we went to Harrods to gaze at the romantic wedding dresses - affordable in our dreams - or to the magnificent food hall, which filled the dreams of my ever-hungry stomach. During one Harrods visit, I had what was a terrifying experience for a young girl when I was apprehended by the security staff! My boss had sent me to buy embroidery canvas and cottons and told me to put it on her account. All I would need to do, she said, was sign for the purchases. This I duly did, knowing nothing about how accounts were operated; the only money matters I had experience of was my loose change of a few pence after fares and paying my Mum each week.

Suddenly, two burly gents were flanking me and asking me to accompany them to the manager's office - I had no idea why. I was bustled into a lift and taken to the top floor, then marched along lavish corridors into a huge room where three men sat behind an enormous desk. They asked me why I had signed for the goods and when I explained they said they had no record of my signature. I was mortified by their hostile manner and felt like a criminal. They questioned me for some time before finally checking with my boss, who said she had not realised my signature had not been registered for the account.

Stanley, the young manager of the LWS, was sent to pick me up and vouch for my honesty. My signature was then recorded for future purchases, but my mortification at being thought a criminal was not improved by the amusement it gave my colleagues when I returned to work!

The people I worked with were interesting and diverse in class and education. Now we talk about the classless society, but however it is arranged I am afraid society will always have different levels. What divides those levels may change over the years; it may be birth, money, education, race, location, religion, style or even physical appearance. As in the animal kingdom, I imagine we will go on sorting ourselves into groups, respecting some, repelling others, creating a hierarchy.

At the LWS, divisions were dictated by education and birth. The owner was from an aristocratic family, some of whom visited us in our workshop. They fully expected to be, and were treated as, superior human beings - although I suspect they had great difficulty in affording their lifestyle. There were two girls who were well educated. One was from a 'good' family who had more money than ability; she fitted the 'genteel' image of the place. The other was an independent woman, quite clever and charming but often irritated by the surroundings. The other occupants of the workroom were my friend from The

Needlewoman and the young male manager, pleasant but a little effeminate.

The characters that passed through our workrooms included Mrs M., the cleaning lady. Her pebble glasses resided half way down her nose and occasionally fell into her bucket of water. Her shoes were always two sizes too large, which meant she had to shuffle along to keep them on. Her back was bent and the broom or mop she carried around rarely seemed to find the corners where the dirt was. Her duster constantly moved over a single piece of furniture while she listened to the latest gossip in the workroom or eavesdropped on our conversations. She was a kind inadequate lady – and very hard up, judging by her appearance. Her white face, framed by jet black hair, and the oversized shoes that she wore left me with the impression of a Minnie Mouse silhouette.

I worked at the LWS for four years until a few months before the birth of my first child, Lee, in September 1959. LWS had its moments, with some enjoyable and amusing memories, but I would never want to go back to that time again, working in such dingy conditions.

CHAPTER SEVEN

RUN-UP TO MARRIAGE

Conventional courtship in the 1950s was so, so different from today. Today's generation would find it all very hard to believe. The simple life reigned supreme and the liberal, more permissive age was still, well, an age away. These were the days when sex before marriage carried a high risk of pregnancy – which would be a major scandal, bringing shame on the family. There was no contraceptive pill, so a thrill was pretty risky. In my fiancé's home, we were not even permitted to hold hands or touch each other in his parents' presence – although, conspicuously, the latter behaved like young lovers. My parents were less repressive and accepted that a modest show of affection was reasonable.

Rod and I enjoyed visits to the cinema, tea on Sunday with our respective parents and occasional nights out with friends. Meals like dinner were rarely eaten out because we could not afford restaurants; instead, we had snacks in coffee bars, fish and chips or sometimes a special treat in an ice cream parlour, with my favourite Knickerbockers Glory. Picnics in the countryside with my fiancé's parents were another treat. We and the picnic were all squeezed into my fiancé's father's little Austin 7 car and off we went without a care in the world.

I began to wish we did not have to commute between our homes so often, especially in the winter when we had a long wait in the cold for buses to go our separate ways for our return journeys home. It became very difficult to say goodbye, and marriage became more and more attractive. The wedding day was not supposed to be for two years, but with the closeness of the promise of marriage we recognised that our need to be with each other and of each other was too strong to wait that long.

In the summer of 1957, Rod asked my father's permission for our marriage on August 23, 1958, much earlier than originally planned. I was still under 21 and so could not marry without my parents' consent. My father reacted badly, regarding me as too young for marriage and telling Rod he was a 'bloody fool.' My parents also had the problem of how to raise the cash for a traditional white wedding. However, not for the first time in my life, my mother came to the rescue. She persuaded my father it was better to allow us to marry for reasons she deemed valid at the time. I guess she thought we might be going too far and we might bring disgrace upon the family. Contraception clinics in those days were only for married women. I have to say with hindsight that my father was probably right. We had very little money, so finding somewhere to live was not going to be easy; I was not particularly domesticated and had led a fairly sheltered life.

Sensibility and dreams are not good bedfellows and as an engaged girl my nesting instincts were coming to the fore. Engagement presents already received included several sets of pillowcases, towels, casseroles, clothes pegs and cake plates. Apart from love, what more did we need? I was so excited at the prospect of becoming a housewife; I dreamed of a little house and garden, and my plans grew every day. My Aunt offered us two rooms - the big front bedroom upstairs and the front room downstairs in her terraced house. We could share the kitchen, which also had the bath in it. The lavatory was next to the coal shed outside at the back of the house. We also put our names down for a council house, which was an unlikely prospect as many families had already waited years to get one.

A year before our marriage, we had heard about a tiny cottage in Fulwich Road, Dartford. It was something like 150 years old and was for sale at £400. (That's right – four HUNDRED pounds!) It had no bath or bathroom and no hot water, and the lavatory was in a separate outhouse in the garden. The cottage was occupied by a tenant, a very independent old lady, in her 80s. Her life was spent in a wheelchair because she had only one leg and the other was paralysed with polio. She looked after herself without help and even managed to decorate her home by putting strips of pasted wallpaper on the end of her broom and then pasting it to the walls. She whitewashed her ceilings by attaching the whitewash brush to her broom. The problem was she had no means of stripping the old wallpaper off so she just papered over the top of the last layer each time.

The front door opened into the small sitting room, from where one door led to a tiny kitchen. This had dark brown painted walls and a shallow earthenware sink; above it, a single cold water tap stuck out from a pipe that ran along the wall. There were no cupboards, just open shelves along the walls for both food and utensils. Buckets beneath the sink held washing in soak. A door led into a very pretty cottage garden. There were two other tiny rooms, both very dark.

We viewed the cottage as an investment, but borrowed half the money from a relative to buy it because we could not get a mortgage - it was too old and in such a poor state of repair. We thought, quite wrongly, that as the tenant was old and frail (and bearing in mind that we did not originally plan to marry for another two years) that her life expectancy could not be very far into the future. We hoped that one day we could make it our home, but we never expected her to move anywhere else during her lifetime. The very small rent she paid helped to pay for essential repairs and agent's fees, but was not enough to repay the loan. Some years later, however, she was offered a council flat and moved out. As we had no money for repairs and around half of the loan was still outstanding, the place was sold without us ever having lived in it!

When we brought our wedding plans forward, we decided to accept my Aunt's offer of rooms - but we were not to know that tragedy was just around the corner for my fiancé's family.

My head was full of wedding plans. The reception was booked, along with the honeymoon in the romantic setting of The Old Mill House, Bickerley, Ringwood in the New Forest. The first night was to be spent at the Charing Cross Hotel in London at a cost of £3.16s.6d; the remaining six days at The Old Mill at a cost of £7.4s.0d. The guest list was begun, argued about, changed and caused a few family feuds before it was finally settled. Planning a formal white wedding seems to cause endless nightmares; perhaps that is why so many people these days shy away from such challenges!

by Barbara Blackston Huntley

On February 20, 1958, I got home from work quite excited because they had told me that for my present I could choose a dinner service at one of London's most famous china shops. I was eagerly awaiting Rod's phone call - I could not call him as his family did not have a telephone and he had to walk to the nearest phone box to ring me. The phone duly rang and I rushed to answer it, only for Rod's words to leave me speechless: 'My Dad is dead!'

I could not believe that my swarthy father-in-law to be, who had never missed a day at school or work until a bout of flu just two weeks ago, was dead.

'What happened?' I eventually managed to ask.

Choking back tears, Rod managed to tell me: 'He came in from the farm for his lunch as usual, went back to work and was laughing with one of his mates when he collapsed and died.'

Neither of us could say anything more and Rod promised he would ring back the next day. The following week passed in a blur until the funeral the day before what would have been 'Blackie's' 57th birthday ('Blackie' was the nickname he was generally known by). I did not attend, staying in Rod's home to prepare the food and drink for the mourners' return.

Rod's mother was devastated; she was now a penniless widow doomed to spend the next 39 years with her memories and increasingly less mobile with arthritis. The family had always lived hand to mouth and had no capital; farm workers did not get a pension. Her only income was her state pension of £3.10s (£3.50) per week. She was 54 (an age at which I retired), but she had to seek work. She found a job two miles away in a grocery shop. She was totally dependent on the local country bus service - and waiting for that bus on wet and windy mornings, with her painful arthritic legs, was very difficult for her.

Rod was worried about her living alone after our marriage as her other son was serving in the RAF. He suggested we might live with her, sharing the rent and household bills. I agreed but my parents didn't think it was a good idea, as they knew I was not a country girl at heart. Rod's Mother was a little reluctant at first, but in the end decided it was a good idea until we had saved a bit more. I did not immediately consider the consequences of moving to a home with no bathroom, a toilet in the garden and only a tiny kitchen with a large butler sink. There was no fridge or even room for one, white washing was boiled in a gas boiler and other washing was done by hand. A kitchen cabinet filled all the remaining space; it had a pull-out flap on which all the food was prepared. However, I was young and in love so of course did not listen to my parents concerns for me living in more primitive conditions. Alas, the conditions I was to live in were the cause of much distress to me later on.

My mother-in-law-to-be wanted our marriage plans to go ahead and so I went off to London to hire a wedding dress. I did not wish to spend future years looking at a dress that I could no longer wear or which became yellow or sad with age. Also, money was tight and hiring one was obviously less costly. I also hired the pink and turquoise dresses for the two bridesmaids. The hire company gave me my veil and head-dress. I was concerned about how to shorten the long pointed sleeve for my polio-shortened right arm. I need not have worried as my mother was told that as long as she did not cut the material she could shorten the sleeve, which she did very efficiently.

Those few months before the wedding were rather strained at times. Emotions collided as my future mother-in-law struggled to cope with her grief at the same time as we were making all our wedding plans. Worse, arguments in both our homes about who should be invited to the wedding were common. By Sunday, May 11, 1958, I had clearly had enough as my diary testifies: 'Tears over our marriage, I don't want to go on!' But on the next day my diary says I bought pale blue undies for my honeymoon!

It seems I was also obsessed at that time by food, as I recorded most of what I ate. I was dieting for the wedding - a practice which was not nearly as common then as it is in today's age of obesity. I suppose I always felt a bit of a freak as most of my girl friends were 'normal' sizes, but I was a size 16 when 10-12 was the average. I think if there were only one piece of advice I could pass on to other girls it would be never ever diet – eat everything in moderation and stay energetic.

After work my time was spent knitting and sewing for my trousseau; much of this involved altering sleeves and hems. We still had no TV, so it was easy to listen to the radio while sewing. I was also excitedly shopping in the lunch hours for clothes for 'going away' on our honeymoon. I recently found a list of items I packed - all very different from what I would pack now. It included:

1 taffeta dress for evening, 2 cotton dresses, 1 flowered skirt, 1 pair white shorts, 1 pair slacks, 4 blouses, 1 swimsuit, 1 cardigan, 3 under-sets in white, pink and blue, 3 pairs of airtex knickers (very romantic, I don't think!), 1 pair cotton panties, 2 roll-ons, 1 bra, 3 pairs fishnet stockings (they must have gone well with the airtex knickers!), 2 night-gowns, 1 housecoat, 1 pair white sandals, black walking shoes, plimsolls and slippers. Accessories included 2 pairs of gloves, 2 hats, a white stole, a mackintosh, 2 handbags, shoe brushes, polish and a duster.

Everything had to be done at weekends and lunch times as I was only allowed two weeks' holiday per year and was saving these for the honeymoon. By July most of the preparations were complete and we bought my wedding ring, a plain wide gold band. A great assortment of casseroles, towels, sheets, pillowcases, tablecloths, tray cloths, tea services and three cruet sets arrived as wedding presents. We attended our respective local churches to hear the banns read. At my church, I had to make a sudden exit with a stomach bug. I hoped this wasn't the Lord's revenge for my move away from regular churchgoing!

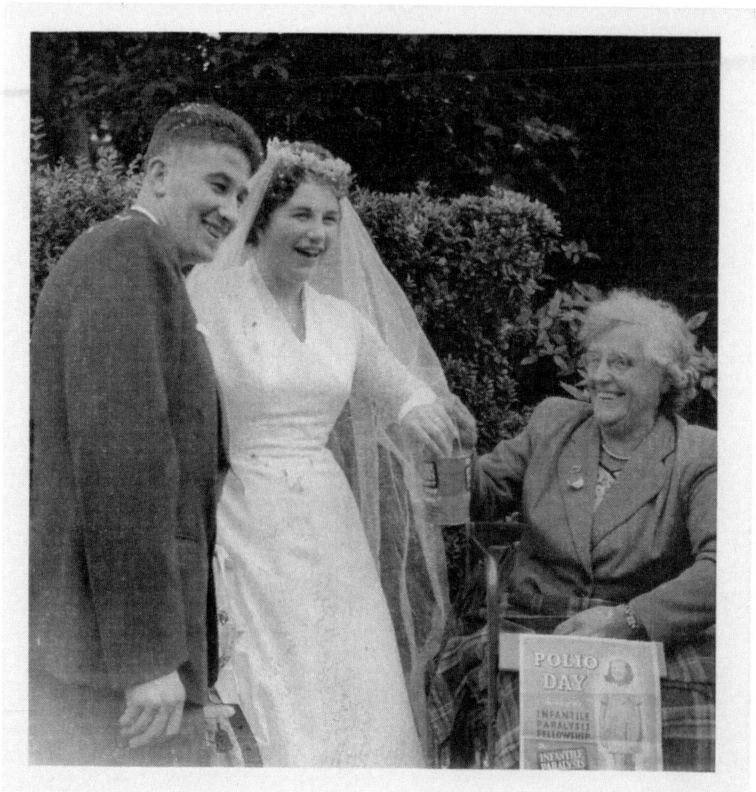

Marriage to Rodney on Polio Flag Day

The collector was Beryl Whiting

23 August 1958

CHAPTER EIGHT

WEDDING AND HONEYMOON

I'm not entirely sure there is such a thing as a "normal wedding and honeymoon," but I can confirm that ours was truly memorable for a variety of reasons, not all of them the usual sort! Indeed, it is the little moments I remember most clearly, rather than all the pomp and ceremony. My wedding day, August 23, 1958, was one of the few days in my life when I was given breakfast in bed, apart from when I was ill. Ours was a traditional white wedding, in a church with my father giving me away (although I did not promise to obey my husband, which was just as well really!). The ceremony was followed by a reception in Acacia Hall, the club premises of Rod's company, at that time known as Burroughs Wellcome.

I remember two great aunts arriving at our home the night before the big day. Both were great characters, but both suffered drunken husbands and were now widows. Aunt Alice's husband was reputed to have urinated in the wardrobe one night after a bout of drinking. Aunt Emma was a great actress; always suffering from pain (real or imaginary is hard to say). Her colourful descriptions of how she managed to dress and undress in the face of such adversity were very entertaining; with face screwed up, very red and distorted, she would say: 'Oh Vilie' which was how she addressed my mother, 'THE PAIN! THE PAIN! You can't imagine how I feel! I didn't think I'd ever get me jumper over me 'ead, I ain't 'ad a wink of sleep in nights, I don't know what I'll do with myself, girl.'

The descriptions of her arthritis grew more detailed and lurid at each visit until one wondered how she ever managed to leave the house. So while she was busy describing her latest symptoms to our wedding guests, I went off to change. My mother said I could dress in the big front bedroom she shared with my father. The bridesmaids dressed in my bedroom. I always wanted to do everything well in advance, so was dressed much too early. Another lifelong problem for me has been the desire to go to the toilet very frequently, but especially when I know it will be out of reach for a long time. When my wedding car arrived, the chauffeur sat patiently smiling in our front room while my bridesmaids went to work with me. They had to assist in holding up my dress and train while all three of us squeezed into our narrow bathroom for me to use the lavatory! It was not easy and prompted much laughter. My Dad had previously had a few qualms about walking down the aisle with me because he said that with his very bent back, my paralysed arm and Rod's paralysed leg we would look like a load of cripples! It had never occurred to me before that he might be quite sensitive about his ankylosing spondylitis.

It was raining when we arrived at the church - St Michaels & All Angels, Wilmington in Dartford. The photographer asked me to stand beneath the lych gate. As I did so, water dripped down the back of my neck and made me stand up sharply, at which point he promptly took his picture. I had not realised he was on my right side. I did not like being photographed from that angle because of my polio arm, but I said nothing.

I remember Rod looking very happy during the ceremony – in stark contrast to his mother. Who remained grief stricken throughout that her husband could not share the day. The church was full of all our relatives and friends and when we came out the sun was shining. This was a lovely moment. I really enjoyed seeing everyone together, chatting and laughing while all the photos were taken.

When we arrived at the gates of Acacia Hall for the reception, we got out of our car to put some money in the tin of a flag-seller because – entirely by chance - it was Polio Flag Day. When we had discovered this coincidence, we thought it would be useful publicity for the Polio Fellowship, we told the local newspaper The Kentish Times and their photographer and reporter came along to record the event – on the front page, no less, of the next edition. Cue our '15 minutes of fame.' The reception was for around 70 people and was generally very jolly. A band played 'Tea for Two', which was the first song we heard being played in Acacia Hall after we got engaged. Rod's Mum was so tearful, though; she hid herself away in the kitchen and refused to join the celebrations. I understood her grief, but was very sad for Rod that his mother could not join in what should have been a very happy day for all concerned.

The whole day flew by, but one little incident I remember occurred after one of my frequent visits to the ladies. As I came out again, I slipped and my size 16 behind crashed to the floor. My legs flew in the air, displaying blue stockings and pink and blue garter, and my elbow went through the lace of my hired dress. All very elegant, I don't think!

We left the reception with several cars following us and honking their horns all the way to Dartford station. On arrival, an officious jobs-worth of a ticket collector was adamant that no-one without a platform ticket should come onto the platform. Not to be outdone, while he was clipping the tickets of travellers, our guests crawled under his arms and onto the platform, where they scrawled "Just Married" in lipstick on the train windows and tied toilet rolls to the door handles! Fortunately, when we arrived in Charing Cross the platform was on the opposite side of the train so the decorations were not visible and we hoped no-one realised we were on our honeymoon - although our new clothes and my pink boater hat could have given us away!

We had booked to spend one night in the Charing Cross Hotel, where our room overlooked the station forecourt. The place appeared very splendid to me, as I had never stayed in such opulence before - now I would probably consider it a bit second rate. The corridors were wider than the rooms we lived in at home; the people we saw all seemed rich and classy. I tried very hard to be a sophisticated young wife. So I was mortified by my new husband's nonchalant behaviour in front of two Arab gentlemen in flowing white robes. Rod had been a smoker for many years, and preferring to roll his own cigarettes rather than buy ready-made. These were very sparsely filled with strands of tobacco, which constantly fell out of the rolled paper, with burning bits of ash and paper sometimes drifting to the floor.

They were smoked to the bitter end, leaving just a tiny stub barely large enough to remove from his mouth. Remove it he did, though, and he then flicked one of these disgusting objects right across the path of the flowing white robes and into an ashtray on the floor of the corridor. I could not believe my eyes. That was the first of what became a tirade of objections to his smoking habits, which remained a big bone of contention between us even after 40 years of marriage. When I die, I won't need to be cremated because I reckon I'll be perfectly smoked! Smoking in the 1950s was entirely acceptable for men, but there were still some taboos for women if they wished to be thought of as ladies. A lady would not smoke in the street and would never leave a cigarette in her mouth. Those who were seen doing such things were regarded as very cheap and uneducated. I did smoke but always tried to follow the socially accepted code.

Our room was probably a little larger than the standard hotel bedrooms of today because there was no en suite bathroom, but we had a large green chamber pot that slotted into a cupboard beneath the washbasin. I would not have fancied being a maid in those days when such vessels had to be emptied for all the guests, especially as rubber gloves were not used.

The first night of our honeymoon was not the stuff of which romantic novels are made. Unfortunately, the pill had not been invented and with nature's sense of humour the time of the month was wrong. Rod had bought a pair of pink leopard skin patterned pyjamas, but he had never worn pyjamas since childhood. After that first night, he never wore them again, either. For most of that first night, we just sat on the deep window-ledge watching the London traffic and the people passing below; so much for an exciting first night of the honeymoon!

Next morning we caught a train to the New Forest. We stayed in a very old Mill House in Ringwood. There was not a straight floorboard in the place. Our room had a very rickety wardrobe that stood on three legs, except when we moved at all, either in bed or out of it – in which case this evil beast banged its fourth leg on the floor remorselessly. If the other hotel residents had not initially realised we were honeymooners, they must have done so soon enough – although I should add that much of the noise related to less exotic actions, such as cleaning our teeth or trying to find a matching pair of socks from the bottom of our suitcases.

Our other problem was the washbasin in the room (again no en suite). If we were washing at the same time as the people in the next room, and the sink plug was removed in one room, the force of the water going down the waste pipe would remove the plug from the washbasin in the adjoining room. This could be very disconcerting! The toilet and bathroom were at the opposite side of the house to our room, along a corridor. The roof sloped down sharply above the toilet so anyone sitting on it suffered a headache if they didn't remember to duck before rising; this was very good for waking you up in the early morning!

Two honeymoon incidents in particular have remained enduring memories. The first was the lady, a fellow guest, who asked me "how I prepared my rice puddings." I didn't have the foggiest idea, but nor did I want to let her know I was a new bride. So I had to say we did not really care for them. It must have looked strange when we tucked into some in the dining room a few days later! The second memorable incident was when we took a long bus ride into the forest and then discovered it returned by an entirely different route and there were no more buses that day. We were reduced to hitch-hiking – and got a very good lift with a friendly tanker driver.

The forest was a magical place and the wild ponies were wonderful creatures. Nothing was commercialised and there were few buildings. The trees, especially the majestic oaks, were magnificent with their late summer foliage. It was a romantic place all right, but we had no transport of our own so were limited to places where we could either walk or get a bus. It rained for much of our week away. Migraine had also somewhat marred the honeymoon for me. Worse, I had developed cystitis and was in a lot of pain. Again, the homecoming was not the stuff of romantic novels. And now the realities of married life were about to hit me, but fortunately I still had a very rosy view of life!

CHAPTER NINE

MARRIED LIFE BEGINS

I did not enjoy the most auspicious of starts to married life. Our worldly possessions were meagre; I was living with my grieving mother-in-law, where home comforts were far fewer than I had been used to in my single state.

Those worldly possessions – Rod's and mine – amounted to £50 in savings and a few wedding presents. These mostly consisted of towels, sheets, two blankets, a candlewick bedspread, seven casseroles, three cruet sets, a bedroom chair, a linen basket, three tea sets, a dinner service, a cake plate, a carving set, and an eight-day clock - but no cuddly toy!

Now I had to tackle the domestic scene. I suppose I was not very well trained for marriage, which in the 1950s still meant putting one's husband first in all things. The most valued women were those who cooked all the meals, kept the house spotless, scrubbed and polished, washed curtains frequently, kept bed linen and tablecloths whiter than white and always had a smile on their faces (or that was how the advertisers saw it).

Husbands were still the major providers of housekeeping money - mine was to be £4 per week for many years to come. They generally chopped wood and carried coal into the house, did the decorating, carved the Sunday joint, mowed the lawn if you had one and did the gardening. If you were lucky, they helped with the washing up occasionally. Mine was a 'new' man because he sometimes vacuum-cleaned as well!

It had been agreed that we would live with my mother-in-law until either the cottage we had bought became available or we had saved the money for a deposit for another place, which then seemed an unlikely prospect. My mother-in-law was generally referred to as Mrs B, which was the way I addressed her before our marriage, as she would not allow me to call her Mum before the ceremony. Nor was it was considered polite to address one's elders by their first names. It seemed strange calling her Mum after our marriage. I eventually got used to it, but it was awkward referring to her dead husband because I had never called him Dad, only Mr B. Now I had to refer to him as Dad, when he was no longer alive - which all seemed very peculiar.

My husband's home was so different from my own; it was the home of a poorly paid farm labourer with two sons. It was a very masculine household which I, as an only child of a father who was not very 'macho', found hard to deal with. I had almost never seen my father even stripped to the waist. Mrs B was a dominant and determined woman, with little time for feminine behaviour; she had to be tough to face up to a very hard life. There were few fripperies in her life and certainly no luxuries. She was a plain cook, Sunday roast swam in fat, and puddings of meat or Spotted Dick were served frequently. Fat and fresh vegetables were the mainstays of the family diet. Bread was served in doorstep slices.

Furnishings were simple, but the rooms were crowded. Numerous old magazines were stored and every available corner or surface had plants standing on them or hanging from them. Dust was always plentiful, as was the mud brought in from the nearby fields. For good measure, the men of the house had all been smokers. There was no bathroom or bath. The back part of the house was an outside toilet and coal hole. The wooden door of the toilet had a large gap at the top and bottom and was freezing in winter. Sitting in contemplation was not advisable in cold weather as one might well have suffered hypothermia! It had its good side, though - it was very effective in sobering up the lads after a night on the town.

The scullery, or kitchen, as it was later called, was about two metres long by one and three quarters wide. It contained a large butler sink with a wooden draining board, a gas cooker, a gas boiler and a large kitchen cupboard. Over the sink was a small Ascot water heater, which provided enough hot water to wash ourselves and the dishes.

This was my first week at home with my new mother-in-law. I had to prove I was domesticated! The tiny kitchen was my new training ground. I had to learn how to light the gas boiler and bring the washing to the boil. Then I had to extract it with a large copper-stick, transfer it into the big butler sink full of cold rinsing water, and then take it into the garden to put through the large iron mangle beside the outside toilet. The rollers were made of hard wood, which had softened somewhat with age. This contraption had to be cleaned before mangling the clothes because it was not protected from the elements. In winter the ice had to be chipped off first. For the rest of the year it was covered in bird droppings, blossom or leaves.

The handle was very heavy to turn, especially when mangling flannelette sheets. Sad to say, one of my early attempts at doing the washing did my reputation as a budding housewife no good at all. I did not realise that only whites could be boiled; coloured items were washed by hand in the sink with water taken from the boiler and cooled when all the whites had been done. I put yellow dusters in the boiler with my husband's white shirts and mother-in-law's white tablecloths. Disaster! Everything came out yellowy grey in colour! Bleach removed the yellow, but they remained slightly grey. The event took a lot of living down; still, my cooking efforts generally were well received, so hopefully that restored my reputation a bit! There was no fridge, so perishable food was bought daily from the village butcher, grocer or greengrocer.

We spent this first week after the honeymoon stacking away the presents we hoped that we could one day use in our own home. Thank-you letters were written and photographs touted among the relatives. After our wedding pictures had been in the local papers, we had a surprise letter from Matron Brown, of West Hill Hospital in Dartford, where Rod and I had been as children with polio. She had been the Sister on the ward when we were both in hospital at the same time; she remembered us and wanted to see us. A visit was arranged and we were all delighted to meet up again; the Matron was very interested to hear how well we had progressed over the years.

That same night, on September 5, 1958, we went to visit Rod's club. A terrible storm blew up so we decided to take a taxi home. When we got there the street was flooded and we had to paddle to get into the house, which was fortunately above the flood level. The newspapers described it as 'The Storm of the Century.' In more ways than one, our honeymoon was well and truly over.

Mrs B decided that it would be better if she did the housekeeping; she would prepare evening meals and I would do lunches when I was at home. The family included Rod's younger brother, Gordon, when he was home on leave from the RAF. We were to give Mrs B my £4 housekeeping money plus £2 for rent and the money for Rod's bus fares to work, which she returned to him daily. I paid my own train, bus and tube fares to work, out of my own wages, and saved the rest.

After marriage I did not work on Mondays, which was when I did all the washing and ironing. In the evenings I sewed, mended or knitted. Sometimes – still with no TV, remember - we played monopoly or lexicon (a game of lettered cards played a bit like scrabble). Rod sometimes played crib with his mother and aunt but I did not like playing cards. At weekends we often visited the many relatives of both our families, sometimes staying with my parents and sleeping on a studio couch in their front room. Rod always went to his rifle club on Thursday evenings and had a drink with his mates. We went rambling with his friends three or four times a year, walking about ten miles through the Kent countryside.

We were all – both families - keen listeners to the radio and avidly tuned in to 'the Archers' every evening. Occasionally there would be a dance at Rod's club or a party in someone's house. At these parties, we played silly games like postman's knock, pass the parcel, or being blindfolded and having to tear the shape of something out of newspaper. I remember when we were supposed to make the shape of an animal and Rod's friend produced a mushroom shape. We all said 'What's that?' and he replied: 'It is part of an animal . . . it's a toad's tool!' Cue roars of laughter. We were a happy bunch of young people and had a lot of fun together.

Less than a month after our marriage, my brother-in-law **Gordon** celebrated his 21st birthday and Mrs B held a party for him in a local hall. I spent the afternoon making sandwiches for the evening and then helped Rod's mother at the party. She had always regarded her younger son as her special baby, so she really wanted the event to go well. I think it did so, with family and friends playing games, dancing and particularly enjoying 'knees up, Mother Brown' in a very boisterous and jolly manner. Everyone collapsed with laughter at the end.

In November, 1958, I came of age (it was 21 then), but as the wedding had taken nearly all our spare cash I could not have a big party. My mother said she would hold a small one in my old home on the Saturday after my birthday. I managed to buy a new dress of royal blue velvet with a swansdown collar, which I thought was really lovely. I made myself a cake and iced it to take to the party. My actual birthday was on a Wednesday and for the first time (and the last, I think) I completed a football coupon. Doing the pools was a national pastime, especially in working class families; it was certainly a great tradition in our two families.

In the evening of my big day, Rod took me to London to see Simple Simon at the Whitehall Theatre, where I think Brian Rix was the star. I don't remember the play, but I do recall going to the Chicken Inn afterwards for supper. My diary merely says it was a wonderful evening.

Rod bought me a portable Singer sewing machine on hire purchase for my birthday. I was so excited and couldn't wait to use it as I could now make my own clothes more easily. I think it was one of the best presents I have ever had. It's certainly the longest lasting and is STILL going strong now, after over 56 years of fairly constant use. I made dresses for the family, trousers for little boys and curtains for my home; I even made my own suits at one time. It remains a very treasured possession and has been used to make fancy dress costumes for my grandchildren. I am still using it for curtains and repairs for my some of my family's items. I haven't yet been asked to make fancy dress clothes for my two great-granddaughters, but you never know!

We were joined by eight friends for my 21st party at my parents' home. I helped Mum prepare the food and we had a great evening. The next Saturday, after enjoying a friend's big party in a hall, I witnessed a horrific tragedy. We were on the train pulling out of Erith station. As I leaned out of the window, waving goodbye to our friends, a man ran alongside, clearly anxious to get on even though the train was picking up speed with every second. I screamed as, to my utter horror, I saw him fall between the platform and the train. His body was repeatedly rolled over as the train sped along and the poor man was ripped to pieces. He was still alive when the train screeched to an emergency stop. With shocked passengers looking on, he was rushed to hospital by ambulance, but died shortly afterwards from his terrible injuries. I was traumatised, but in those days we got over things alone and more quickly than today, when counselling seems to be advocated for everyone.

I grew up a lot in my first few months of marriage. I realised that I had been very protected by my parents and that managing to make ends meet was no easy task. I had always been encouraged to save, but I had not had to budget for a family. I very soon discovered the problems money, or rather the lack of it, can bring. Nonetheless, by the end of 1958, I was still quite starry-eyed - dreaming about one day having my own home and beautiful little babies to fill it – but in the meantime the difficulties of living with my mother-in-law were dawning. I was homesick, I was a town girl living in the countryside, and life was simple and basic. My new home was nowhere near as clean and comfortable as that of my parents because Mrs B did not believe that housework was of any importance. Illness was to be endured without fuss and in silence; she was a very tough lady. My husband shared her views, which had stemmed from poverty and his need of constant hospital treatment and visits to outpatient clinics - always an all-day job then.

There had been little time for sentiment. Rod, in 16 years, had needed 15 operations because of his polio and he had spent over a year in one hospital. Although I came to understand these views, I found life very hard to take at times. Rod was kind, but did not understand my feelings, so I generally kept them to myself. In particular, I kept them from my parents, who were not happy about the way I was living.

My first Christmas as a married woman was spent in my husband's home. My father would not allow me away from home on Christmas Day before I married as he felt it was a family affair, so this was the first time, apart from when I was in hospital with polio, that I had my Christmas dinner elsewhere. Because it was my Mother-in laws first Christmas as a widow the day was spent quietly, but we did play a few games. We all got along fine together, but I missed my own family and thought about them a lot.

Then, after Christmas, it was party time with friends who had married earlier in 1958 and who had their own bungalow. I suppose I was quite envious of them in this respect; I wondered how long it would be before we could save enough to have a roof of our own. About this time, my brother-in-law had finished his service with the RAF. This meant even less privacy for us.

In late January, 1959, I got up feeling rather sick and generally unwell. That may have been responsible for a small incident that caused much amusement to my new family, giving rise to much teasing. As I had such a long journey to my work in Knightsbridge, I had to get up at about 5.40 am each workday. I always dressed in the dark to avoid disturbing Rod, who did not get up until 7.15 am. I went down to the kitchen sink to wash and returned quietly upstairs to dress. Then I went downstairs again, made Rod's sandwiches for his lunch and slipped out of the house into the winter darkness, still trying hard not to disturb anyone. I caught a bus to the station, then had a 45-minute train journey to London, followed by a walk to the tube to get to South Kensington, from where I had a 10-minute walk to my work.

The lights on the tube were fairly bright and I noticed people looking at me somewhat oddly. I just stared back until I was about to get up from my seat, when I glanced at my feet. Oh Lord! The sight embarrassed me for the rest of the day; on one foot was a shiny black pointed toe shoe and on the other was a brown shoe with a round toe and in need of a polish. I could do nothing about it, as I had no money to buy another pair. All day I either hopped from one leg to the other or tried to hide one leg under my skirt, hoping my predicament was not obvious to all the clients. Fortunately, the trains were crowded on the way home and so there was little opportunity for anyone to study my feet until I got to the bus stop for the last leg of my journey. I was very glad when at last I got home and could stop impersonating a stork!

Meanwhile, the nausea of the previous day returned and I began to suspect that I was pregnant. A few days later, I was coming home from work when I suffered very severe pains, vomiting and bleeding. I was taken by the next door neighbour to see my lady doctor who said I was having a threatened miscarriage and must go straight to bed. This was the start of a very difficult time. I desperately wanted to save my baby, but I could not keep any food or drink down and rapidly became dehydrated, losing a stone in weight. I was also suffering constant pain and was taken to hospital, where they thought I would spontaneously abort the baby.

I remember vividly the first meal I had there - tripe cooked in milk. The white crinkley rubber-looking cow's stomach was cut into small squares, but it made me feel sick just to look at it. The nurses insisted it was good for me and persuaded me to try it. I think they regretted their action as very soon after the first mouthful they had to clear up the results. I had warned them! I am glad to say the meal was not repeated during my ten-day stay. Much of the time was spent lying flat on my back, but eventually I managed to keep most food down. Then the doctor said I could go home. This was a great relief as my ward had been full of geriatric patients. I sympathised with them, but their plight was very depressing for me when I was still not sure whether I would have a miscarriage.

On my first day back home, Valentine's Day, I was on top of the world. Although we had not planned a baby so soon, and had hoped to have our own home first, the thought that I might have lost the baby made me want it more than ever. I was excited and already making plans. Mrs B had kept my husband's baby basket that was rather dusty and aged-looking, but I planned to line it and make a frill to cover it. We had so little money that we had to be resourceful. Alas, within 24 hours of my return home, the euphoria had passed and the constant sickness returned. I became more depressed than ever and extremely tired. Just two-and-a-half weeks later, I was back in hospital for another five days, but there was very little they could do. I think they partly assessed me as living in stressful conditions at home, which I suppose was true, but I did not want the family to know how I felt.

My parents read between the lines and often invited us to stay. My father had just bought a new Ford Popular car, which was quite exciting for Mum and Dad; they really enjoyed taking us out in the country for a ride at weekends. I had to give up travelling to London every day, but I did some work at home and just went up to London once a week to return or collect work. On one of these trips, I bought the material to make myself a maternity dress, smocks and a summer coat. I had very little money to spare for clothes, so I had to make them myself, although my Mum bought me a maternity skirt. Clothes always had to be practical and suitable to wear afterwards. My first winter coat after marriage had to last me for 16 years. Fashion was something I read about in magazines, but could not really afford; it was a dream for the future. Fortunately, although it sometimes took me a long time, I could sew quite well, even though I could not raise my right arm due to the paralysis, my fingers worked a little but not my thumb.

My days at this time when at home were spent working from 8 am to 12 noon. Then I would cook lunch, followed by sewing in the afternoons, and then knitting for the baby or reading in the evenings. One evening a week I might go with Rod to his club or to the meetings of the IPF (Infantile Paralysis Fellowship now the British Polio Fellowship), where we met other polio victims. Sometimes there was entertainment or maybe games like beetle drives, cards, darts; otherwise we just enjoyed a natter and a cuppa. Occasionally, we arranged a concert, made the costumes out of crepe paper and rehearsed in our own homes. I particularly remember producing 'The King and I', where we involved all the children of the polio victims or their families. It was very colourful and the children's singing was warmly applauded.

On Sundays Rod and I would often walk in the fields and orchards at the back of his home, taking with us Mum B's little dog. These were very happy days when we could enjoy each other's company without family around - when we could sit at the edge of a cornfield in summer with a bottle of lemonade and talk about what life would be like when the baby arrived and when hopefully we had saved enough to get a home of our own. Not in my wildest dreams did I ever imagine that we would one day own a refrigerator, two cars, two televisions, a computer (I hadn't even heard the word 'computer' then, anyway!), or go any further than Calais or be able to financially assist our families.

I suffered sickness throughout my pregnancy. In June the weather was very hot and the visits to the hospital for exercises and antenatal care seemed to bring on particularly bad attacks and severe exhaustion. I nearly always walked from Wilmington to West Hill Hospital in Dartford, the last stage being up the very steep hill from the town. I could not afford the bus fares when we were saving so hard for a home of our own and a one-week holiday at a holiday camp.

Most afternoons while we were away were spent resting in bed because I felt so ill. I had grown to huge proportions and looked like I was carrying a baby elephant rather than merely being six months pregnant with a child. Each morning I avidly ate my breakfast and then rushed (well as fast as my mountainous body would allow) out of the dining room, along a corridor where all the cleaning ladies stood aside for me, through the ballroom and into the toilets where my breakfast ended up each day. The cleaning ladies shouted out to each other along my route as I dashed past them

'Here she comes, clear the way! Morning dear, no better then?' Needless to say I was unable to answer them!

We had seen an old terraced house for sale at £1,250 in mid-May, 1959, and decided to try and buy it. We paid a deposit and set the wheels in motion to obtain a mortgage from the local council, who at that time lent money over a 30-year period, and we found a solicitor. Once more I became very excited, planning the baby's bedroom, imagining myself as the perfect housewife in my own home. I window-shopped for curtains and furniture. We planned the decorating and layout of the rooms.

We had to wait two months for the council's decision - until the full council met to determine mortgage applications. In the middle of July, we were rejected. We just did not have enough money for the work on the house that needed to be done before the council would grant the full mortgage. I was heartbroken and cried, my plans all dashed; I would have to go on living with my in-laws. It was very unlikely we would be granted a council house as whole families waited on the list in overcrowded conditions for many years. I loved my husband, but I now knew that my father had been right. We should have waited to marry until we could have afforded a home, or at least a flat.

CHAPTER TEN

MOTHERHOOD

My diary at the time says it was "the best experience of my life" – the birth of our baby son, Lee Rodney, at 6.45 am on September 30, 1959. Certainly, the experience – plus the build-up and all the consequences – TRANSFORMED our lives!

I left work in July and went up to London to say farewell to my colleagues. I felt sad, but was thrilled to receive a beautiful hand-made shawl from my friend Jean. Baby clothes then were mostly hand-made and I set to work making long nightgowns for the baby on my new sewing machine. Each gown was long enough to come well below baby's feet and had a drawstring at the bottom; sleeves were also long enough to have drawstrings around the wrists, which were pulled down over baby's hands at night to keep out the cold. The garments were made out of cream flannel.

The knitted layette comprised numerous matinee jackets with matching bootees and bonnets, leggings for cold weather, coats and mittens. I had made some myself, but knitting was a fairly slow process for me because of the polio, I could only move the left knitting needle but I had developed my own method just holding the right needle in a rigid state. It got quicker as my pregnant bump increased and I had somewhere to rest my paralysed arm! I was grateful to all the friends and relatives who produced so many of the garments. Coloured baby clothes were just becoming accepted (previously most were white); pale yellow or green were knitted before birth as there was no way of knowing the baby's gender. After birth, pale blue or pink knitted garments were often made, as appropriate for a boy or girl.

I look at the lovely little garments produced nowadays; they are so colourful and easy to care for that it makes life seem easier, but we did not have to follow fashion. The pressures upon us were quite different. The biggest pressure, as it still is, was finding enough money for food and accommodation. But in those days we were also judged on the whiteness of our sheets, towels and nappies hanging on the washing line, the cleanliness of our children and the state of our homes. Were the floors and furniture highly polished? Were the surfaces dusted . . . were our husbands' meals ready on the table when they came home from work? Good mothers had well-rounded babies in spotlessly clean prams and used washing powder that got the clothes 'whiter than white.' They were dedicated to husband and children and did not "work" unless misfortune had left them without money.

One task I really enjoyed was making a new frill for the baby basket that my husband had used as a baby. Money was now very tight and I was glad to accept my mother-in-law's offer of the basket. I bought white seersucker material with little floral sprigs in pink and blue on it. This looked very pretty when finished and served well enough. Mum B and I made a mattress and blankets for it. Much of my time was spent sewing, knitting, crocheting and preparing everything for the baby. I tried to walk a little every day, usually accompanied by Mum B and her dog. It was a very hot summer and in the last months of pregnancy I was exhausted.

My greatest hunger pangs came at night, when I would raid the larder for anything going. There was a glut of plums that year and they were very cheap, so I bought several pounds and devoured them around 3 am every night, my sins there for all to see each morning with the pile of pips on the bedside cabinet. Also on my nocturnal diet were large slabs of home-made fruitcake, with my husband being reasonably tolerant of the resultant crumbs in the bed. He did get rather annoyed, though, when his sleep was disturbed one night by me crunching my way through the only thing I could find to eat - a large stick of hard seaside rock.

On August 23, we celebrated our first wedding anniversary. Rod gave me a bouquet of carnations and a red rose. My father gave me a summer shawl for the baby; I received flowers from my mother, while Mum B and my brother-in-law gave us some soup bowls. This was a very happy day in the middle of a difficult time emotionally for me. The child I was carrying was extremely active, my weight had increased enormously (I guess the fruitcake and rock had not helped), and I could not sleep. The constant hot weather was making life difficult, especially as the house had no bath. The sickness I had suffered in the early months of pregnancy returned. My doctor prescribed phenobarbitone tablets - unthinkable now, when we know how drugs can damage the unborn. I have wondered many times if these were the cause of later problems for me.

The baby was due on September 18, but seemed in no hurry. I began to feel happier and more positive. When baby had still not arrived by September 24, the hospital decided to keep me in and try to get things moving – but still with no joy until five days later. Rod visited me in the evening and just before he left I felt a pain - the labour had begun at last. I shook with excitement! There was also fear – could I cope with the pain? Would the baby be okay? There was no going back; life would never be the same again. Rod did not know what was happening to me; fathers were not expected to attend the birth and were generally regarded as a nuisance by maternity staff if they hung around the maternity ward. I would have liked Rod to know I was in labour, but there was no telephone at home. So I just had to accept he would not be nearby for this unique experience.

Our beautiful baby son weighed 8lb 1oz; he was well rounded with dark curly hair. He was gorgeous and sucked his thumb as he lay in his cradle. I was euphoric, as if I were the only person in the world feeling this way. Rod rang the next morning from a phone box – still not knowing he was a dad! He asked how I was and when the nurse told him we were both doing well he was very surprised and had to ask what sex the baby was. When he heard, he was so excited that he punched his friend, who was sharing the phone box, shouting 'it's a boy!' The friend was almost knocked off his feet and out of the phone box!

Women then were 'churched' before leaving hospital a few days after the birth. We were taken to the hospital chapel and blessed. I remember the vicar praying that Rod's 'quiver be filled with arrows' - a reference, I believe, to his ability to get me pregnant again! This was not the best timing for such a sentiment, with me still sore from just giving birth to the first one! I rather irreverently had to stifle my giggles at this point.

Ten days after the birth, I went home a proud mother. Many who did not know us well were curious as to whether my baby was 'all right,' as both his parents had polio. Their ignorance infuriated me, especially when it was obvious that they were looking my baby over as he lay in his pram.

Lee was christened a few days before his first Christmas, in the gown in which his grandmother had been christened. The angelic look and behaviour were deceptive portents for the future, though.

My mother-in-law had declared vehemently before Lee's birth that she was not having him dumped upon her while we went out, but that soon changed. Whether it was his charm or not, I don't know, but it did not take her long to volunteer her babysitting services. Lee became her very special grandson for the rest of her life, although she had four more grandchildren and five great-grandchildren. The relationship with Lee remained special, maybe because he helped her come out of mourning and maybe because he was born while we shared her home.

Shortly after that first Christmas, we felt that we had to have our own space; the little cottage was not really suited to all our needs. The front door opened into the small front room, which was only just about big enough for the three-piece suite, side table and large pram that had to stand there. The back living room, also quite small, contained a tiled fireplace, a heavy dining table and four dining chairs covered in leather, two wooden carver chairs, a large sideboard, a sewing box on legs, plants and all the things for daily living. Food had to be prepared for cooking on the dining table, as there was so little room in the kitchen. Here, too, Lee was bathed and powdered generously with talcum powder. In fact, the table was the centre of most activity - dressmaking, mending, curtain-making, household repairs (the tool kit was kept in the coalhole or the large cupboard under the stairs).

The staircase went up between the front room and living room. The cupboard opening into the living room was an absolute glory hole. It had tins of food, bottled fruit, Christmas puddings, important papers, tools, gas and electric meters, raincoats, wellingtons, old newspapers and magazines, tins of paint, tins of buttons and badges - and much more.

Rod and I decided that if my Aunt was still willing we would accept the offer of two rooms in her house. This left us with the problem of how to tell Mum B. It was not easy and there were many tears, but I think she finally accepted that we had to break away at some time. We left on January 16, 1960, moving to my parents' home in Erith. We stayed there until we had decorated and furnished the rooms we were to rent in my Aunt's home just across the road. My Aunt offered us the large front room and even larger bedroom. There were no power points and the rooms had not been decorated for many years. An electrician friend wired the front room so that we could have a kettle, toaster and radio.

We got very excited about buying our first furniture and decorations. We chose a grey pattern of small bricks with ivy trailing over it for the wallpaper. The curtains were bright red on one side and black on the other; they were fairly dominant in the room, as the sash windows were quite long. Red and black was our colour scheme; the carpet square we chose was also mainly red with a little black, as were the plastic backs and seats of the four dining chairs we bought. The table was a very heavy drop leaf affair with a cupboard right through the middle and a drawer at each side. Cupboard space was of primary importance. Friends gave us a very old brown kitchen cabinet. We bought two fireside chairs with wooden arms and we were given my Grandmother's old wooden fireside chair and her washstand with its marble top. We used this as a worktop where we placed the shiny new electric kettle and toaster. That completed our downstairs room.

Upstairs we had the large front bedroom to share with our small son, but had little money left for furniture or decoration. The only new item we bought was a divan double bed with a straight wooden headboard bent slightly round at each end, very much in the style of the late 1950s or early '60s. The only other furniture was baby's cot, a Lloyd Loom chair and linen basket, which were wedding presents, one of Grandma's dining chairs and her chest of drawers. There was no wardrobe, but a cupboard in the recess beside the fireplace in which to keep our clothes. We could not afford to decorate the room; it remained as it had been in 1954 when Grandma died.

I was elated to move in; at last I was to a certain extent mistress of my own two-roomed home, although we still had to share the kitchen with its bath and the outside lavatory and coal hole. The arrangement was that during the week I would cook my family's evening meal at 6 pm before my Aunt and her friend returned from their jobs in London. This seemed to work well enough and I felt as if I had a great deal more freedom; we could now invite friends and family to tea without asking permission or receiving censure. Friends rarely came to dinner as the budget did not run to big meals, but tea on Saturday or Sunday was more common.

My cousin Iris and her husband lived in the same road, in rooms with her widowed father. We had been very close as children, but had not seen each other for many years. After our joint grandmother's death, there had been a quarrel between her seven children and the family divided into two factions. My cousin and I were the daughters of opposing sides, so we were not permitted to meet or communicate with each after the quarrel.

We met one day while out shopping and were really pleased to see each other again. We both agreed the quarrel had been very silly and there was no reason for the next generation to carry on the feud, which had begun over the ownership of a tin bath hanging on the fence of my grandmother's back yard. My mother and Aunt had both claimed they had bought it and so should inherit it on Grandma's death! The resulting argument meant that for five years half the family had not spoken to the other half.

Iris and I decided to meet on Wednesday afternoons to share a cup of tea and cakes from our local bakery. These were usually very gooey, a keenly anticipated indulgence we both enjoyed while discussing our problems and the dreams that one day we might have our own homes, with our own kitchens and maybe even a proper bathroom. My cousin gave birth to a son in the August after we had moved to my Aunt's home, and we decided to celebrate. One Wednesday afternoon we chose to forego the tea and instead open a bottle of home-made elderberry wine I had been given. Unfortunately, the small glass we started with got topped up and as we did not think it was very strong we decided on a second glass. Luckily, my cousin only lived a few houses further up the road because it appeared the pram with her son in it had developed wonky wheels by the time she went home!

My little son was now very round and plump with a shock of blond curls. He was the apple of his grandparents' eyes, while my father frequently came home from work at lunchtime to see him. Lee wolfed up everything I gave him plus some things he was not meant to eat, such as coal from the coalscuttle beside the fire! Once, I had to leave the room for a moment after I had dressed him in red rompers, white shirt and red bow tie, all ready to go out. While I was gone, he found his father's ash tray and ate all the cigarette ends he found in it. In the process, he ruined his angelic pristine appearance, presenting me with a yellow-stained, ash-strewn urchin. Needless to say, I was a little late for my appointment!

Most times, though, he was a happy baby with a smile that lit up the room. He chattered incessantly in his own way and loved to watch people in the street outside. Some of his first words were 'Whose zat? Who is it?' - repeated over and over again until it drove us mad. I always tried to play with him in the afternoons before tea. Bedtime was soon after his Dad came home at 6 pm. With no TV, there were no distractions and life followed a fairly orderly pattern. We read a bit in the evenings or listened to the radio, I made my clothes, mended or prepared meals for the next day. Mending clothes was a never-ending task; men's shirts were for best occasions when new, but when collars and cuffs became frayed they were removed by unpicking all the stitches, turned over and stitched back on, and they were then working shirts. When the reverse side frayed, they became gardening or painting shirts. Sheets that had become worn in the centre were cut through the middle and the outsides were turned 'sides to middle' and stitched up the centre. When too worn for the double bed, the best bit was used to make a single sheet; when that was too worn, the best bit could make a cot sheet, under pillowcase or handkerchiefs.

Socks had to be darned, trouser pockets renewed and most cardigans or jumpers were hand-knitted. This was a slow process for me because of my arm, but I always had a great sense of achievement when I finished a garment. There was no mistaking my shortcomings, though, when I began knitting a pair of leggings before my son was born and finally finished them well after the birth of my second child! Mostly, I relied on the kindness of my mother and her next-door neighbour, an elderly widow, who knitted far more expertly than I did, and finished the children's garments well before they became adults. I once spent a whole year knitting a waistcoat for my father. This was definitely not my forte!

CHAPTER ELEVEN

OUR FIRST REAL HOME

We had been very grateful for my Aunt's rooms and our relationship with her and her friend was always very good – but of course our driving ambition remained a home of our own. At last, the opportunity came when the occupant of the cottage Rod had bought before our marriage – that incredibly independent elderly lady in her wheelchair - was rehoused by the local council at her request.

The cottage had to be sold on because we had no money to repair it; the transaction would give us a deposit to buy a house. Rod sold it for £1,400, paid off the remaining debt to his Aunt and, after legal fees we had £1,000 for that deposit. We thought this was an enormous amount; we had never seen a four-figure cheque before and kept looking at it before paying it into the bank. I was tremendously excited and anticipated no problems with such a big deposit.

We started gazing into estate agents' windows and finally found our dream semi-detached house in Dartford. It was £3,000. We viewed it, then confidently marched off to the estate agents to confirm that we wished to purchase. The agent was all charm until he asked how much my husband earned. 'About £12 a week, but we've got a big deposit of £1,000,' he said.

The agent gave him his poor deluded fool look; the charm disappeared like silk from a smooth body to be replaced by syrupy condescension. 'I'll just work it out for you, Sir, but I don't think you will get a mortgage of £2,000.' He duly presented the shattering conclusion. I just could not believe my dream had fallen at the first hurdle; it seemed Rod would need to earn at least £18 a week even to be considered. Such a leap in pay was unlikely in the near future. We went home disconsolate, knowing our sights must be set lower.

With Lee approaching his first birthday, we so wanted to have another child before he was too much older, but our living conditions were not sufficient. We searched on and found a semi-detached house about half a mile from where we lived, in Hurst Road, Erith, at £2,800. We heard that the local council was offering 30-year mortgages to young people whose wages were not enough for a 25-year mortgage. When we asked the agent about it, he said my husband's wages were still not quite high enough, but Rod had found an extra job one evening a week teaching scientific glassblowing to trainee laboratory technicians at a local technical college. This was bringing in another £78 per year, and it did the trick! He scraped through and got his mortgage, to be repaid at £13 a month. We were overjoyed, we couldn't believe that at last we would have some privacy in our marriage; we could decide what we wanted to do without always having to consider its effect on the rest of the household and whether they might be listening. At last we could be a proper couple living under our own roof.

We moved into our new home on December 10, 1960, on a freezing cold day with ice coating the steps down to the garden at the back of the house where the overflow pipe from the bathroom had dripped; in my heart, though, it was midsummer!

Our new home in Lesney Park was built around 1934; it was on top of a hill and had about 200 feet of garden. Upstairs were two very large bedrooms, a box room and a bathroom. Downstairs we had a large lounge with a high wooden fireplace with an inset oval mirror. There were huge folding doors that opened into a fair-sized dining room with a high wooden fireplace, French doors to the garden and a serving hatch to the kitchen, which was long and narrow with an evil-smelling coke boiler. Heating was with coal, from a bunker in the garden. There was a covered area for a small car, but no way could we afford one of those! The house had no carpets; linoleum covered the hall floor, one bedroom and part of the dining room. The kitchen floor had lino tiles; the rest of the house was bare boards. We had no money for carpets or furniture apart from the little we had when we were in rooms. Fortunately, the rooms had picture rails and we hung our clothes from them until someone took pity on us and gave us an ancient wardrobe.

The previous owners of the house had not yet got their new home and asked if they might store their furniture in our lounge until they found somewhere to live. We did not mind as we had nothing to put in the room anyway, but we did not realise it would be about three months before they finally collected it.

Because we had only just moved in, we had Christmas in my parents' home with their next door neighbour - who asked me when my baby was due!

'I am not pregnant that I know of!' I replied in amazement.

'My dear, you ARE - I can see it in your eyes,' she insisted.

I was, in fact, just a few weeks pregnant - but had yet not realised this, what with moving house and all the associated problems.

So my wish to avoid a big gap between my children's ages had been granted, but there was so much work to do in the house with decorating and making curtains that I thought I would have little time to prepare for a new member of the family. Still, I already had lots of baby clothes, and as babies of both sexes were dressed similarly I did not need to worry too much. My big fear was that money would not stretch to meet all our needs, but fortunately I had been brought up to be very frugal and to waste nothing. I made my son's trousers out of old tweed skirts or bought remnants of material in the market for a few shillings. This helped the budget, but buying shoes was a problem as my son's feet grew amazingly fast.

I still had only £4 a week housekeeping money for food, household items and any personal needs. About £1 to £1.50 went on groceries and around 36p on bakery items, £1.00 on meat and 85p for dairy products; anything left over was used for sewing materials and shoes. The baker called every day except Sunday and the milkman every day including Sunday. From them, most fresh foods were bought as we had no fridge. I wanted to save up to buy one as we lived at least 20 minutes' walk from the shops - so fresh food had to be purchased daily in hot weather. I could not bear to throw food away.

Our meals were very different from those I prepare now. A joint was always bought for Sunday lunch and the leftover meat served cold on Monday, with leftover vegetables fried as 'bubble and squeak'. Any bone left-over went into soup on Wednesday with a marrowbone, which the butcher sold me for 3d (1½p) and lots of vegetables. Meals on Thursday, Friday and Saturday were most likely to be shepherd's pie, corn beef (very cheap then) or sausages. Once in a while, though, it would be lamb or pork chops, or a piece of fresh fish. Some vegetables and fruit we grew in our garden. Breakfast on Saturdays and Sundays was our treat with bacon rolls or bacon, egg, mushrooms and baked beans.

A meal out would probably be fish and chips. Very seldom did we eat out, but parties in our own homes were common. We held one such party on the second Christmas after moving into our new home. Both our families and friends were there - from my husband's grandfather, who was in his 80s, to the smallest babies. Although we had been given a radiogram (a huge wooden edifice) by a friend of Mrs B, we did not rely on music for our entertainment. I don't think we stopped laughing the whole time as we played numerous games. These included 'the Honeymoon,' with unsuspecting guests sent out of the room and called in one at a time, blindfolded, to sit on a chair in the centre of the room. The people inside the room were told to sit in silence, but anything that the person on the central chair said was supposed to be the comments made on the first night of their honeymoon. Comments would come out like:

'What am I supposed to do?'

'Are you going to say something?'

'Do I have to keep the blindfold on?'

'If you don't say something I'll sing or jump up and down!'

The victim was given one minute of this treatment before being told what was going on before the next guest was brought in.

Another game involved two plates. Out of sight of the guests, we would blacken the bottom of one with smoke from a candle. The room would be darkened. The person knowing the game held a torch in one hand and the clean plate in the other, and the other guest was given the blackened plate, with the clean side towards her or him. They were told to hold the plate up in front of themselves and copy the actions of the person sitting opposite them with the torch shining on the bottom of the clean plate. That person then drew their finger across the plate and then across their face, down their cheeks, nose and forehead. The poor unsuspecting guest then ended up with a very black face and could not understand when we said the game was finished. We would say something like 'Oh, it wasn't quite right; we'll do it properly later.' It was only when the poor victim looked in a mirror that they saw their blackened face - prompting great hoots of laughter.

We would also form two teams to play a bit of a saucy game. We would play a record than suddenly stop the music. The first member of each team then had to remove an item of clothing and lay it on the floor to stretch the longest distance; this was then repeated until all the members of the team had dropped out because they were not prepared to remove anything more. The team with the longest line of clothes were the winners (ties and belts were very useful items). My maiden Aunty was considered to be very daring when she removed her dress and stood in her long petticoat, bra, girdle and knickers! It caused a lot of giggling, but by this time the little ones were asleep and so this was considered harmless fun. However, poor Aunty was never to be allowed to forget her indiscretion; she was frequently teased about it.

Life was hard, but people did not complain too much. As today, we moaned about the Government and the difficulties of making ends meet, but we clung to the belief that we would one day have a better life. Work was an ethic, not just a means to an end; if one had a caring employer, loyalty on both sides was the likely reward. I did not need a charter to tell me how to behave because my upbringing generally had taught me good manners, politeness and respect for authority; I honestly believed my hard work would be rewarded. Without those things, people could be sacked on the spot; there was no such thing as an unfair dismissal procedure. If you weren't wanted, you were sent packing - but at least it was easier to find other work.

Perhaps the less pleasant changes to workers' lives have come about because loyalty now seems to have little value, jobs are rarely for life and financial considerations appear to rule everything from birth to death. Cynicism seems to have replaced the sense of fun that existed when I was younger.

At least Rod and I regarded his job as secure. So as long as I managed the housekeeping properly, we could pay the mortgage each month. I had no washing machine, but I was given an electric boiler and my mother-in-law bought us a belated wedding present of a spin-dryer. This pleased me very much as most of the water was squeezed out of the nappies before they went out on the washing line. It was always a joy to see a line of white sheets and nappies blowing in the wind high up on a single washing line strung between two posts (I hate modern circular washing lines). In the winter, when they could not be dried outside, and with no central heating, clothes were dried on a clothes-horse before the fire.

We still had no TV, although many people we knew now did - but not our parents, or most of our friends. When Lee had gone to bed, I did the things I found difficult to do during the day because he was such a hyperactive little boy. Each week I made a batch of small fruit cakes. I cut out clothes, sewed or did my accounts as I ran a catalogue amongst family and friends. This earned me commission that I saved for my refrigerator or other needs. One item we really needed was a stair-carpet as my toddler son would clomp up and down the bare wooden stairs very noisily - but for nine months we could not afford one. We managed to decorate the hallway with bamboo-patterned wallpaper. This was a difficult job because of the long drop down the staircase from the top of the landing. Rod balanced with his good leg on the window-ledge of the landing window and the polio leg on the banister along the top landing passage whilst I, in a very pregnant state, leaned over the staircase to hand him the paper and tools to hang it. My heart was in my mouth, but he succeeded. We saved up and eventually bought the cheapest Indian cotton carpet we could find to deaden the noise of going up or down stairs.

by Barbara Blackston Huntley

Most of our furniture was second hand; it was a jigsaw puzzle that came together over a long period. When my cousin emigrated to Australia, we bought their bedroom suite and TV. Hooray! At last we had somewhere to hang our clothes and had drawers in the dressing table for jumpers and underwear. For me it was exciting and the very ancient wardrobe we had been given before was moved to the spare room.

I was preparing for my second child, but did not have the time to plan and think about it as I had for our first. I found the task of running a whole house, bringing up a toddler and carrying another child quite daunting, especially with Lee such a handful. One morning, returning from a shopping trip, I undid the strap on his pushchair and carried some of my shopping to the kitchen. When I turned round, he had emptied a large bag of flour onto the coconut front door mat - all done with the sweetest of smiles! Another time, while I was hanging out the washing, he squeezed the washing up liquid all over the kitchen floor and as I came through the door my feet went from under me. I caught the handle of the overhanging grill pan as I fell to the floor. The pan overturned, hitting me on the head, and I landed hard on my behind. His angelic face did pucker somewhat when I gave an almighty roar of fright and frustration. I could not stand up it was so slippery. With shovel and rag, I removed the mess, ending up with the cleanest kitchen floor in the street!

Then there was the time Lee stood up in his cot and discovered he could pull whole sheets of wallpaper off the wall. I could barely see him beneath the mess, but once more that grin surfaced. Another time, he climbed on to the back of a chair in the lounge, slipped and crashed through the window cutting his chin. But the most frightening episode came after the birth of my second child, when he put a hairpin into a power point. This blew him backwards, burning the pin into his hand. I grabbed the baby I was feeding, dropped them both into the pram, and ran to the local hospital a few streets away. Lee was none the worse for his shock and won over all the nurses with his mop of blonde hair and that beautiful smile! I never knew what he would do next. I was always afraid of leaving the room because of his antics, but most of what he did seemed to be out of curiosity. I was always relieved when bedtime came round and his angelic head rested on the pillow. Come 6 am, though, the little brain was preparing Mum's torture for another day!

CHAPTER TWELVE

OUR SECOND CHILD

Sad to say, I never forgave Rod for missing the births of both our children – for not sharing either of the two most important events in our married life. This time – for the arrival of our daughter Krista – Brands Hatch got in the way. Rod always went there to marshal for the motor racing on the August Bank Holiday. Before he left, I felt unwell and told him the baby would arrive that day. He said it wouldn't, suspecting I was trying to keep him away from his beloved racing. I insisted this was the day because of how I felt, but he went anyway. I was almost right as that day I went into labour but had no way of contacting my husband. He did not reach the hospital until some 3 hours later. He was worried and very apologetic. I was still in labour but I hardly spoke to him and he went home quite quickly saying he would ring in the morning. Krista came into the world the next day 4.30 am on Tuesday, August 8, 1961; once again Rod was not present.

We gave her just the one name as we could think of no other that sounded quite right with it; also, extra names always seemed a nuisance when completing forms. When Krista grew up, though, she wished she had a second name. She was born with very dark, straight hair and very pale, beautiful ice-blue eyes. Her weight was similar to her brother's at birth, but she was quite different in looks; she was a contented and undemanding baby. Lee loved her dearly from the start, but any attention she received was very much noticed by him; anyone saying what a lovely baby she was would be told: 'I'm lovely, too!'

Lee was now two months from his second birthday and greatly enjoyed being with people. As I could not attend the first birthday party for my cousin's son, my mother dropped him off there. As the front door opened, I'm told he rushed across the threshold into the room where the other children were shyly clinging to parents or playing quietly. Not Lee. Without any malice, he promptly rushed around the room – and knocked over most of the children in his haste to get to the toys and food! Quiet moments were never again to be the order of the day when he was around – unless, that is, he was fast asleep. I was so pleased that my little girl had been born on the birthday of my cousin's son. It proved a most economic arrangement for future children's parties as we held them on alternate years!

Life eventually settled down to a pattern where I could cope with the home and the children. I still tried to be the 'model housewife,' polishing floors and furniture zealously. I did not always succeed, though, and my mother would sometimes come in offering to help clear up. 'I know you are doing your best dear,' she would say, 'but things do get out of hand with the children, I know. I will just give the cooker a clean for you.'

She meant well and I was very sensitive - but her offers made me feel totally inadequate. I think many of the problems that came between us stemmed from the fact that I was an only child and she could not forget that my arm was partially paralysed; she constantly felt that I needed help. With other children to distract her attention, it would have been better for me. She had no more children because of my polio arm and the war, but in a way I felt I was to blame for her not having the bigger family which she always said she would have liked. I was so glad that I had two children, although they were never great companions in childhood.

Looking after the garden in our new home was quite demanding; fortunately, Rod took care of it most of the time. The children loved it as it was divided into different areas, with a lawn at the top, flowerbeds in the middle, vegetables and fruit trees and a roughly grassed area at the bottom amongst the fruit trees and bushes. We put a swing in one of the trees. It was also a good place to play games and have great bonfires on Guy Fawkes Night. On November 5, family and friends would come around; I would make a huge pot of marrowbone and vegetable soup and fill the oven with large jacket potatoes baked until the skins were really crisp. Everyone 'oohed' and 'aahed' over the fireworks, while the bonfire lit up the gardens, crackling and spitting showers of sparks into the night air. The bonfire was a good place to get rid of unwanted items, the neighbours often contributing. It was always a wondrous occasion for all the children over two years old; they were far less sophisticated than today's children. We found that under two years the fireworks tended to frighten them, so they were usually put to bed. The Guy Fawkes tradition was kept up by my family and later by my brother-in-law's family for many years; it was always eagerly anticipated. On cold nights, it was good to come in from the garden, remove all our thick outer garments and tuck in to the steaming bowls of soup.

On the home front, money began to get even tighter and I sought part-time evening work. I got a job in a cardboard box factory, from 6:00 pm to 9:30 pm, four nights a week. I went out as Rod came home from his work. My father generally fetched Rod from the station and took me to work each evening. My job involved stripping the waste from piles of cartons designed and printed on flat sheets of card that were partially punched out. The waste was thrown onto a moving belt; then the cartons were made up by the day shift. My work was very hard on the fingers, making them sore. The factory was very cold in winter and we took it in turns to make a cup of tea half way through the evening. Unknown to me, this was against the rules as we worked less than four hours.

Another of my tasks was to stick pieces of brown glued paper over the inside corners of cardboard boxes. This was soul-destroying and very boring, so I tried to think about the money I would save for all the things we needed to finish furnishing our home. Maybe we could get a new bed for our son because we had only an old second hand one but needed a spare for when Mum B came to stay. I slogged away for three months. It was not only boring but also quite taxing because the waste-stripping really needed strength in both hands. I could grip things with the fingers of my right hand, but had no strength or power in my arm to keep the work in place. I dared not mention this to anyone for fear of being sacked. Nor did I want sympathy or help from anyone else because that would have been unfair on them. I usually stood at the end of the working line to the right, to avoid others noticing my struggles.

Then disaster struck one day when it was my turn to make the tea. There were about 12 of us in the shift, including the foreman, so the tea was made in a large enamel pot and taken to a bench in the middle of the factory. On my way from the kitchen with this very heavy pot, I caught one foot in a loop of string lying on the floor. The loop tightened and tripped me up. I tried to hold the teapot up but fell over with the scalding hot tea emptying itself over my good left arm. Someone sent for an ambulance while someone else covered the burned arm with a headscarf. I was wearing a cardigan and watch. The cardigan had retained the heat and the watch was embedded in the now blistering arm. The ambulance seemingly took an age to arrive and the pain was intense, but finally I was taken to hospital; the cardigan and watch were removed and I was placed on a trolley to await attention.

I had picked a poor night for a mishap; there had been a bad traffic accident, killing one man and seriously injuring others. Their needs were greater than mine and I waited two hours for further attention, with the blisters turning huge; they hung like great sacks from my arm. Eventually the doctors and a nurse came and slit them open, allowing all the fluid to escape, and dressed the arm from shoulder to finger tips. I was devastated! How was I to cope with two small children, let alone the shopping and cleaning?

This hospital was some distance from my home - a ten-minute walk and then a bus ride. The arm needed to be dressed every day, but I could not get to the hospital alone because I could not manage the buses with the children even before the accident - I could not fold the push chair and hold a baby at the same time. Rod had no car and my parents could not accompany me, as they were both at work, and we could not afford taxis. Fortunately, the hospital agreed that in the circumstances my arm could be dressed in the local cottage hospital, which was walking distance from my home.

My husband realised that I was now helpless and asked his employers whether he might take some holiday, as we could not afford the loss of earnings. Burroughs Wellcome, as it then was, came up trumps and granted him compassionate leave with pay. It lasted a month, but I was so grateful he was there at home to look after the children.

The whole experience was shattering for me because I had never been so helpless. I could not wash or dress myself or handle my personal hygiene. Just having my face washed felt very undignified. I thought a great deal about people who are totally paralysed. Their indignity and frustration must be extremely hard to bear and the situation must seem impossible if you also cannot communicate your thoughts and feelings. Sometimes my poor husband suffered from my irritation at being so hampered. I don't think I could have been very easy to live with at this time!

The healed physical scars remain on my arm to this day, but the mental fear of being helpless goes even deeper and will never heal. I eventually returned to my evening job, but my heart was no longer in it and I resigned after a month - much to the relief of my employers, I suspect.

Krista grew into a quiet child who would play happily if left alone, but her energetic brother would not allow this if he was present. Sometimes I felt more like a referee than a mum; do all siblings constantly fall out? Krista loved her books and never tore them, whereas Lee had no time for them; he loved only things with wheels. Lee had to pull everything to bits to see how it worked; he was naturally curious about the physical world. He would argue about everything, but most of all about bedtime. Lee was a total extrovert, Krista an introvert, somewhat shy and lacking in confidence. Each child was a wonder and a worry to me for different reasons. I loved them both so much but could not believe the totally different characters that my husband and I had conceived in these two children. It made their upbringing very hard because each child needed a totally different method to bring out the best in them. I did what I thought was best for each one, but many times I have wondered if I failed one or both of them. Still, I have always been glad that I had the chance to be a mother, and the joys have mostly outweighed the traumas and worries.

If there was one piece of advice I could give to prospective mums, I would say: remember you may also be having a terrible tot, a stroppy seven-year-old, a rebellious teenager . . . and it doesn't end there. When they take a partner, they may come back to you with their problems, not least insolvency. If you can support them through all those stages, listen with empathy to all their problems, accept being asked for advice but rarely expected to give it, accept that you will be thought old-fashioned and out of touch as they grow older, the kindest and sweetest Mum when they need a babysitter for their children and finally patronised in your old age, then you will make a perfect mother! Fortunately, in some ways we are totally unprepared for what may be our lot when we have a child, but most mums seem to get by even if we are not all model mothers.

Generally, I was lucky with healthy children, although even the normal childhood illnesses can be traumatic. When Krista was almost two, there was a bout of measles doing the rounds. Her eyes and nose started to run and she began coughing - I thought the spots would not be long behind. None came, even though she screamed at the light and the cough got so bad she began choking and had to be held forward, gasping for breath. She ate nothing but oranges and her weight fell sharply. The doctor came every day, sometimes twice, and said she must be kept in semi-darkness and accompanied night and day in a warm room. Her cot was brought into the dining room, where we could keep the fire going; brown paper was placed around the lamp shade to reduce the light and the curtains were kept tightly drawn.

At night I laid a mattress on the floor beside her cot and the moment she coughed I would jump to make sure she continued breathing. For the rest of the time, she laid exhausted and motionless, night and day. I dared not let my husband do the night shift because he slept so heavily and would not have heard her coughing (he never even heard alarm clocks). I was very worried. The doctor prescribed penicillin and at last the rash appeared; Krista had lost seven pounds in weight and was a pale shadow of the chubby little lass we had before her illness. She gradually recovered and I got my first night of exhausted sleep back in my own bed. Rod stayed downstairs with her; I remained very nervous, but finally she was restored to full health.

Away from health issues, I saw a newspaper advertisement for a refrigerator for sale at a lower price than those I had previously seen. Such things were very expensive when compared with the cost of white goods today. I discussed it with Rod and we drew on our savings to buy it. I was so excited. Now I could buy fresh food for several days at a time . . . no more milk with wet towels over it in saucers of water in the summer, no more bacon going maggoty in the larder, no more discovering a bluebottle fly had laid eggs on the meat before you could cook it. Unfortunately, there was no room for this wonderful invention in my small kitchen. So we ran some power to the larder under the stairs and put it in there. For the first few days, I kept opening the larder door just to look at it - I was so proud of it.

My next acquisition was the very latest in washing machines, a twin tub. Washing machines had been like electric boilers, but with an agitator inside and a wringer on the back, but mostly only the well-off could afford them. Now the new machines had one tub with an agitator and one which was a spinner to remove the water from the clothes. This one was a very efficient machine and lasted me 14 years. As women were beginning to go out to work more, this was very high on their list of priorities.

I did not have a vacuum cleaner when we moved into our own home; it was not too important because I only had a square of carpet for the dining room and for that I used a hand-operated carpet sweeper. An aunt eventually gave me a very decrepit old Goblin vacuum cleaner, which seemed to have less effect than the sweeper in removing whatever the family dropped on the carpet. Mostly I just had mats, which were thrown out of the French doors at the back or out of the bedroom windows. They were then hung over the washing line and beaten very hard with the yard broom or my hand brush, brushed off and returned to the house when all the other cleaning in the room was finished. The lino around the mats was polished every fortnight and the kitchen floor was scrubbed on hands and knees every week and then coated with a liquid shine.

The staircase was washed down every week, as were window ledges indoors. The hearth was cleared of ashes every morning in winter and the fire lit with yesterday's newspaper, chopped wood and small pieces of coal. Sometimes embers still burned from the night before and after removing the ash the fire could be rekindled for the new day. The kitchen boiler was loathed by Rod and me; its only use was to heat the water and keep the kitchen warm. It gave out the most dreadful choking fumes and it always seemed to go out just when we most needed hot water. I began to feel the thing had a grudge against me; I regarded it as my enemy in the corner of the kitchen. My cooker had two ovens, one for normal to high temperatures and one for long slow cooking. I found this really useful as I loved to make things like cakes and casseroles at the same time or roast potatoes in one and slow-cook meat in the other.

All the shopkeepers knew me quite well and I had little chats with them. I took my list into the grocer on Friday morning and he delivered the order on Friday night. I bought fresh meat for the weekend and fresh vegetables; the only frozen food was an occasional treat – a block of ice cream wrapped in thick newspaper for the 20-minute walk home.

Rather than a phone of our own, we had an extension of my parents' phone about a mile away. It was little known at the time that this could be done, but as my father was a telephone engineer he was aware of these things. The advantage was that only one rental fee was paid; the phone was switched through to my home during the day when my parents were working and switched back to them at night and weekends. It cost nothing for us to talk to each other for we merely wound a little handle on a black box, which gave a ring on the other's extension. The downside was that sometimes my parents went to work and forgot to switch it through to me, which meant I could not make or receive any calls. But we could never have afforded our own phone, so this was a great boon to us.

My cousin and I still met for our Wednesday afternoon gossip and cakes, but these were more often now the home-made variety. My cousin had moved to the 13th floor of a council flat in Erith. It had a wonderful view across the Thames and surrounding area, the town, the railway and all the local factories. She had a second son born in the flat. With two children each and at least a one-and-a-half mile walk at the slow pace of our eldest children, we more often than not had lunch on our alternate visits to each other's homes.

Life had settled down for us both and I suppose I thought of my cousin more as a sister. So it was a big shock when she told me she was emigrating to Australia under the £10 scheme. Families went on a four-week journey by ship to Australia at the time when the Australian government was keen to attract skilled workers. I was so upset the day we all said goodbye; I felt sure I would never see her again.

CHAPTER THIRTEEN

MOVING ON

Time was flying, as it does, and before I knew it my first little baby was a schoolboy! It meant I had a bit more time to enjoy Krista's company, but I quickly learnt that Lee was opening up a new front for his hyperactivity, namely the school classroom, with his teacher remarking on his energetic nature.

His first day at school was probably also the last on which all elements of his new school uniform looked the way they did when purchased. From then on, his socks were always down round his ankles, the shoes were scuffed, with laces undone, the cap peak was at right angles to his face, and his blazer trailed along the ground. Paint and ink seemed to have an affinity with his white shirts, as did glue and mud. Knees were regularly bloodied. He was just about everything you would imagine a boy to be. Anything mechanical was his heart's desire and if it made a very loud noise so much the better.

When I had taken him in on that first day to Normandy Primary School in Fairford Avenue, Barnehurst, Kent I was relieved to think that maybe his constant energy could now be directed to better uses than I had managed. I felt quite guilty that I seemed to be the only mother who was not shedding tears over parting company with her little darling for a few hours. Likewise, he was one of the few children who sped into the class without a second look back at me.

I did look forward, though, to hearing how his first day had gone, as I went to collect him from the classroom. I asked his teacher – which was a mistake! 'Ah, Mrs Blackston, yes, well . . . ' she began ominously (in a tone I would come to recognise throughout his schooldays). 'I had 36 things in my classroom for the children to do and Lee had done them all within the first half hour; he is a very energetic child, isn't he!' After that, I avoided too much contact with his teacher. I guessed that her few grey hairs multiplied enormously through having charge of my cheerful, enquiring son.

In the meantime, I taught Krista nursery rhymes and read and sang to her, but unfortunately we were a very unmusical family and I had a voice more akin to a frog crossed with a concrete mixer. Whether she was tone deaf or what, I don't know, but she certainly enjoyed my raucous noises and would ask me to sing again. This did my ego the world of good, but anyone else unlucky enough to be within earshot of my singing would cringe and cover their ears. So I tried not to be within range of others when I performed an aria or accompanied a song on the radio.

In the autumn, Lee caught a very bad cold, which turned to bronchitis. He was quite ill and was violently sick. I called the doctor, who seemed to take ages examining him. He discovered that my son had a heart murmur and would need to see a heart specialist. I was very concerned, but it seems a great many people do have this problem, very often without even realising it.

As the festive season approached, I decided we would have a really good family Christmas. We invited my mother-in-law, her father and sister, Rod's brother and his wife and their two small sons, my parents and some friends. I had already made Christmas puddings and on November 6, 1965, I was making the cake one evening. I was thoroughly enjoying all the smells of cooking around me. I was thinking what a good time we could give to all the children, Lee aged 6, Krista, 4, and my two nephews, Tracy, 2, and Glenn, nearly a year old.

Suddenly there was a knock on the front door – and the mood was shattered. Gordon and Chris - Rod's brother and his wife - were standing there with their youngest son in their arms. 'Where's Tracy?' I asked.

'He's dead!' my sister-in-law sobbed.

'Oh my God, what happened?' Rod and I both said.

'He's drowned in a fish pond,' my in-laws managed to blurt out.

They had recently moved to a new farm, where Rod's brother was a cowman and his wife was to help clean the farmhouse for the farmer and his wife. Because she had only just started in her new job, my sister-in-law was not familiar with the layout of the gardens. As she cleaned her son, Tracy walked out of the back door unnoticed. She missed him within a moment and went looking for him – leading to the nightmare discovery of her little boy lying face down in the farmer's fish pond. All efforts to revive him, by his father and the ambulance crew, were unsuccessful. The water in the pond had been icy cold.

Total devastation gripped our whole family. Tracy was a blonde, curly-haired, active little lad of just two years and five months. Just a few weeks earlier, he had been rushing around my house, giggling uncontrollably. How could such an awful thing happen? Not only was it terribly traumatic for the parents, it was particularly distressing for my mother-in-law because she had now lost both her husband and one of her beloved grandchildren. Life sometimes seems unspeakably cruel.

There had to be a post-mortem and an inquest. It was discovered that, not only had my nephew died from drowning, he had a very severe heart defect in which his heart had partially hardened. There was no cure for this. He would not have been expected to live beyond the age of five. It was a minuscule crumb of comfort to think his death was very quick and not drawn out, as it might well have been otherwise. When you suffer something traumatic, it feels as if you can never laugh or enjoy life again. But it's also true that, over time, the human spirit seems to recover. The loved one never departs from our hearts, but we move them into a different place. I suppose the religious call it Heaven, but I prefer to think of it as their spirit within me.

The news of my nephew gave me a dreadful jolt because it also made me wonder whether my own son's heart murmur was something more sinister - that there might be a hereditary element. However, I was reassured by a hospital consultant that there was no such link and that Lee would probably grow out of it, which appears to have been the case. Shortly after this dreadful event, my sister-in-law discovered she was unexpectedly pregnant. Of course, this child would never take Tracy's place, but a new life had come into being almost at the same time as his brother's death. Was it an omen? A new baby meant hope for the future.

Around this time, Rod's maiden Aunt Elsie, known to both our families as just "Aunty," had discovered a bungalow for sale in Dartford. She knew the owners and had explained that my husband and I both had polio and a bungalow would be better for us.

We viewed the bungalow and it seemed quite small after our large house and garden. It had three bedrooms, two of which were a bit smaller than our main bedrooms. The other one was bigger than our box room. There was no dining room, but the kitchen was bigger than ours, with room for a small table. The lounge was quite a reasonable size. The garden was much shorter but wider.

We were struggling to pay the rates on our large house; it was cold and cost a fortune to heat. The garden was a very big problem to keep under control. We decided to sell and buy the bungalow. Deep down I didn't want to go, but I knew it was practical for my husband with his paralysed leg so I agreed to move. The sale of our first real home was to haunt me for a long time, though. For many, many years, I sometimes dreamt I was back there. It will always hold a special place in my heart.

It was very difficult to find a buyer for our first home, but after seven months we sold it for £4,750, buying our new one for £4,800. The bungalow was built in 1932 and had been changed very little when we moved in May 1966. There were very few power points, no cupboards in the bedrooms, and the decorations were not to our taste. Ancient gas fires adorned the corners of two bedrooms. The only other heating was a 1950s gas fire in the lounge. The boiler was similar to the one we had left behind, but not so evil-smelling! There was no garage, but we did not have a car anyway so that did not matter too much. There was a big square lawn for the children to play on and I could easily see them from the kitchen. Everywhere was flat; I missed the steps that made the garden at our former home in Lesney Park more interesting, but this was safer. The bungalow's large hallway was covered in dark brown wood panelling, which I disliked intensely. It was one of the first things to go.

Life was chaotic for a few weeks, but it soon settled into a pattern of what is considered normal for any family with young children struggling to make ends meet whilst trying to save enough to work on a new home. Rod was happy to be back in Dartford, within walking distance of his work and closer to his family. At least my parents had a car, so they could visit us quite easily. Lee and Krista soon got to know children who lived around the close where our bungalow stood. Lee, though, preferred to wander and could often be found on or near building sites or garages, which all seemed to fascinate him. This was a big worry for me.

Now seven, he quickly developed a passion for watching the building of the road from the Dartford Tunnel. Our home was very close to the bridge over the new road and we could stand on it and watch the men using huge scraper trucks to scoop out the great expanse of chalk beneath the bridge. The approach to a single tunnel already existed, but the major road connecting it to what many years later became the M25 Southbound was only just being built.

Then it happened - one day I could not find Lee. I searched frantically. From that bridge, I saw, far below, the dark silhouette of a driver in an enormous scraper against the shining white chalk - with my son held in his lap and his hands on the huge steering wheel. I gasped and shouted, but of course could not be heard against the great din of the machines. It was not a safe place for a small boy and how he had got there I had no idea. I waved furiously. I eventually caught the eye of one of the other drivers below; I waved, pointed and gesticulated madly. At last, it dawned on someone that I wanted my child, and to my immense relief he was returned in one piece. I was very angry with him, warning him of dire punishment if he ever went there again - but he always regarded workmen as his friends. He seemed to be able to persuade all sorts of people to let him have a go at doing adult jobs.

As well as putting the fear of God into me, his exploits were also downright embarrassing. One day I was quietly working in my kitchen when there was a knock on the back door. 'Morning Missus,' said a very dirty workman. 'Your boy said you'd be filling our kettle for us.' This man had come from a site at the corner of our road, where they were building bungalows. Lee was helping them stack bricks and had indeed sent one of them to me. I lacked the heart to say no when, each morning the exercise was repeated with one or other of the builders turning up on my doorstep for their water. What my elderly neighbours made of this, I do not know; they watched all the comings and goings through their net curtains and were always aware of whatever went on in the neighbourhood, night or day.

Another of Lee's wanderings almost led to me calling the police. He was told to be in by 4:00 pm as we were going out. At 4.15 pm I went to look for him, searching every local building site and the parks and garages without success. Rod was not at home and by 6 pm I was returning home in tears. Then, as I crossed the tunnel road bridge, I saw my son walking up a footpath from a lay-by far below. I yelled 'Lee!' He looked up with a happy grin on his face and ran towards me.

'Where have you been? You're a very naughty boy!' I said angrily.

'I've been in that caravan, down there,' he pointed down to the lay-by where a caravan still stood with a car. 'Those people broke down and the man wanted to know where there was a garage so I took him to show him, and he took me back to the caravan and the lady in there gave me some cake and lemonade.'

The story seemed genuine enough, but I gave him a lecture on talking to strangers, with particularly strong words about going into strangers' vehicles, only for Lee to reply: 'But Mummy, they weren't strangers, they were my friends, they were nice.'

How do you explain to a child what constitutes a friend, and besides, are friends always safer than strangers? Somehow I think we as parents had given our children the view that strangers are evil, unpleasant people and friends were nice smiley people, with no "middle ground." I hated to disillusion them. Sometimes it seems very hard even for adults to be sure of who can be trusted.

My sister-in-law, was expecting her baby at the end of the July after we had moved into our bungalow in May. I was most concerned for her, after the loss of her son. I did not want to leave my new home so soon after moving there, but I felt I should help her care for her other son during the last stages of her pregnancy and when the new baby arrived. They had moved away from the farm where their eldest son had died; the memories were just too painful. They now lived in one of a pair of cottages on a farm in Petersfield. It was a lovely area with fields and trees all around - very green and very luscious countryside. My brother-in-law was responsible for the entire dairy herd.

My sister-in-law wrote to tell me that the hospital said the baby might be born earlier than expected. This left me with a problem as Lee had only just started at his new primary school. If the baby came when expected, he would not have missed much, but in the event I was asked to go at the beginning of July. I decided to go earlier and teach him myself for the last few weeks of term. Krista was not starting school until September, so there was no problem there.

Our stay, lasting six weeks, turned out to be very hard work. The children loved it, with so many interesting places to play and make camps. Food could be eaten outside in the sunshine or in the tent that we made for them from old polythene sheets.

For me it was not so good. My nephew developed mumps shortly after I arrived and my two children then caught it. I will not forget the tweedy country doctor who came to see them. He told me: 'Watch the boys' testicles, Mother!' I had no idea why he said that – (I did find out later that mumps can cause infertility if the testicles swell) - and was too embarrassed to ask. However, between watching testicles and doing housework, I managed to make my nephew a pair of trousers out of an old skirt and go to market to buy fresh provisions.

I would do the shopping when my brother-in-law took male calves to market for slaughter. On the first trip, I cried my eyes out because we took a beautiful small black calf with huge brown doleful eyes. He constantly licked my cheek and mooed in my ear. I was convinced he knew his fate and I was very upset; it seemed so cruel. My soft attitude to country life was the cause of much amusement to the farming people around!

Another disturbing incident was when the gamekeeper next door brought back two rabbits he had killed for our dinner. I was amazed when he gave them to me with their fur still on; I had never skinned a rabbit before and had no idea how to start. I waited for my brother-in-law to come home; I suppose I felt quite squeamish, but I did not want to be laughed at. So when he said he would skin them in the outhouse, I said I would watch. I wished I hadn't.

The ears were held firmly and the skin was cut down the underside from throat to belly. Milk flowed over the bench; the rabbit had been a mother who was still obviously suckling her young. I squealed in horror and ran from the outhouse. I could not waste the food, though, without greatly offending the family, and of course it wouldn't have done any good to have binned the animal. I prepared a casserole with a heavy heart. I was very reluctant to eat the meal - yet I had eaten rabbit many times before. The gamekeeper also brought us pigeons, but I did not witness their plucking. I merely used the breasts with bacon to make a casserole. I did not particularly enjoy that, either, because the preparation reminded me of another unpleasant incident. Some time earlier, in another visit to the country, a colleague of my husband had given him some pigeons which he brought home for me to cook. They were just as they were when shot. The dead eyes made my stomach turn but, ever mindful that food must not be wasted; I got out my "Good Housekeeping" book to see how to prepare them. I argued with Rod as to which one of us should cut off the heads. The argument lasted for some time until I jumped up in anger, grabbed the carving knife and chopped off the head of one. The most appalling smell came out because I had chopped straight through the crop, which was full of brussel sprout remains. This time the pigeons did go straight into the dustbin - or I might well have thrown up!

CHAPTER FOURTEEN

HECTIC TIMES

I love the countryside – but I am definitely not a countrywoman. The endless invasion of the house by mud when the weather was wet and by dust when it was dry was a great nuisance that I never came to terms with – and I hated the smell of cow dung that seemed to hang around the whole place. Any chance that I would become endeared to cows evaporated with two unforgettable incidents at the farm.

First, I had to take a message to my brother-in-law, who was doing the milking. I had just bathed and changed into a clean summer dress; it would not take me too long to run down to the cowshed. I opened the door and peered inside. I shouted to my brother-in-law, but he could not hear me with the din of the milking machines. I ventured in, screwing up my nose at the smell; I walked further down the shed and mistakenly stood behind a particularly large animal. At that moment, a great stream of green muck was emitted with immense force from her rear, covering me – clean dress and all - from shoulders to feet. As Queen Victoria said: "We are not amused!" But it did give the family many laughs during the retelling over the following months.

The second incident came when my sister-in-law was in the maternity hospital giving birth to her third son. All three children in my care had caught mumps and were confined to the house. My seven-year-old son hated being indoors. It had rained heavily, but the sun had come out and the trees were dripping with sparkling droplets of water. Blades of long grass in the fields opposite twinkled in the sunlight, but as I looked out I saw brown and white cows trampling everywhere. They were in the road and in other fields where they were not supposed to be. The wretched animals had escaped from the field they were put in. No-one was at home apart from the children; my brother-in-law had gone to market. I ran frantically from the house - forgetting I was only wearing sandals - and banged on the gamekeeper's door. He was not there, but his wife said she would phone a neighbouring farm for help. I tried to shoo the cows into a single field, but it was hopeless. The wet grass was up to my knees and I got soaked, ruining my sandals. I heard a commotion and looked back to the house to see my two children hanging out of the bedroom window shouting encouragement. I was terrified they might fall to the garden below as I rushed around in a field opposite the house. Much to my relief, just as I was thinking 'what the hell do I do now?', a farm hand from the next farm came by on his bicycle. He went for assistance and the animals were finally rounded up.

One more incident at this time sticks in my mind. It was rather spooky and I cannot reasonably explain it. My husband came to stay one weekend and we decided to take a walk together. We had been apart for some three weeks, missing each other a lot. An hour or two to ourselves was a precious break, especially as it was a warm and pleasant day. We went along the lane beneath a place called The Ridge in Peterfield and then up through the woods and fields to the top to look at the view. We held hands and chatted happily, but fell more silent as we started to climb The Ridge. About two thirds of the way up, I suddenly froze. I had a terrible feeling of evil all around me. I was petrified, in a panic and glued to the spot, fearing to go any further; I knew with total certainty that I must go back! There was nothing to see, but I was cold and the various greens of the woods around me seemed to darken and become very oppressive.

'What is the matter?' Rod asked.

'I can't go on!' I said

'Why ever not?'

'There is a dreadful evil atmosphere here, can't you feel it?'

'No' he laughed.

He tried in vain to get me to carry on, but I was adamant. He accepted that I was feeling real terror and we hastened back down the hill. He could not understand what had happened and nor could I; I have never had such a feeling of evil before or since. When we returned to the house, Rod told my brother and sister-in-law about it. They agreed it was mighty odd and later mentioned it to the farmer and his wife - who told them about a local legend.

It seemed that many years before, in Victorian times, there was a story of a local man who believed his wife had been unfaithful. He suggested a ride out one day in his open carriage. They rode almost to the top of The Ridge and he got out, leaving his wife inside. Then he whipped up the horses; they careered down the hill, overturning the carriage and killing his wife. Whether this is true or not, I have no idea. Whether mine was a paranormal experience connected to the incident is beyond me. Generally, I do not believe in such things. I prefer to think they are caused by the sometimes strange tricks the human brain can play on us. I only know that on the day of our walk I could not voluntarily have taken one more step up that hill.

When my sister-in-law brought home her new son, I was free to go home. I had been away for six long weeks and was desperate to start work on sorting out my new bungalow. Although my in-laws had been grateful for my help, I am sure they were happy to have their privacy again. I had been very homesick and longing to get back to suburbia.

My Krista was due to start school in September, 1966, and she was very much looking forward to this. Pinafore dresses were made, uniform items purchased and name tags ordered and sewn into all her clothes. I loved needlework, but the hand sewing was a slow process for me so I really had to get cracking. On Krista's first school day, I was so proud as I photographed her outside our new home, wearing the grey pinafore dress I had made and her first school shirt with over-long sleeves to allow for growing. Her brother was also proud to be in charge as the schoolboy who knew the ropes. He had a protective attitude towards her and, although they fought like cat and dog at home, they always stood up for each other at school.

We had managed to get rid of some of our oldest second-hand furniture before leaving our Lesney Park home. We had bought two red moquette covered armchairs, which were not new but a vast improvement on the old leatherette chairs we had in our lounge previously. The newer chairs were intended to match with a red studio couch given to us by my parents; this doubled as a spare bed for visitors. We bought a small green and white gingham-checked table with pull-out leaves for the kitchen where we would now eat our meals. This was designed to match the green enamelled sink with its surrounding green cotton curtain. Under the window was a range of ancient, grey-painted, wooden cupboards, their top being the work surface covered in a Fablon material which had been damaged by knife cuts. In the corner of the kitchen was an old larder with a small window at the top.

After my big house, the whole bungalow seemed quite cramped, but it was certainly cheaper to run. We settled down quite quickly and the children seemed happy in their school. I missed having a telephone in the house; our former arrangement was not possible as we were too far from my parents' home. We certainly could not afford the rental. Luckily, there was a public telephone box just around the corner, but I missed having chats with my parents. We did not get a phone of our own installed until June, 1973, some six years after we moved in. Most communication was by letter or postcard. The postal service was very good; a local letter posted first post invariably arrived second post. The postman was generally regarded as a friend and tended to have a regular round. We did not have first or second class stamps; a letter cost 4d (less than 2p) in September, 1966.

I began preparing yearly accounts and these show that in the year 1966 we spent in present decimal terms:

Electricity	£16.50
Gas	£28.00
Coal	£28.10
Rates	£51.25
Mortgage	£167.00

My husband's wages now were about £73.50 per month after stoppages. Our mortgage had increased because it was over 25 years instead of the previous 30-year term. Budgeting was hard, but I managed because grandparents often bought things for the children. They never had new toys from us except at Christmas or birthdays. Our son's main playthings were Leggo, which was added to each year, an Action Man, and small cars or lorries. For our daughter, it was a doll, a tea service or books. A few bigger things were bought second-hand, like a twin doll's pram and a train set.

The children made a great deal of their own entertainment. Living in what was effectively a circular close, with another small close leading from it, there were plenty of places for them to play outside. There were very few cars then, so during the day the street was fairly empty and children rode bikes, go-carts or scooters around the circle. Mostly, though, a crowd of them would gather in the garden for a picnic, making a camp or dressing up in Mum's old clothes. Sometimes they had an old tin bath filled with water for paddling and splashing around. For playthings there were wooden spoons, a bucket, cocoa tins, old patty tins filled with mud for imaginary cakes, old cake tins, stones, bits of wood and anything else they could lay their hands on when Mum wasn't looking. The noise could be deafening - or sometimes too quiet for my peace of mind. It occasionally felt as if I was providing a field kitchen for an army, I was referee at some spectacular fights, too; I was the first aider for broken heads, cut fingers and grazed knees. As time went on, I added hairdressing, washing and bathing facilities to avoid children going home in so much of a mess that they would be unrecognisable to their doting parents. Much later I even became an agony aunt to a few of the local children and sometimes even their parents. Two children of different families had particular problems, although both were in trouble at different times and one took drugs, I believed they were both good at heart and would always chat to me. Difficult home circumstances had driven them to fight the world that had given them a poor deal. They were both welcome in my home and were always very polite to me even when they grew up.

The children liked to watch television (black and white) when they had their tea, with Blue Peter and Dr Who among the favourites. Krista was terrified of The Daleks in Dr Who and would watch the programme from behind the sofa with her head half hidden and one eye peeping out at the screen through her fingers. If things got really scary, she would rush out of the lounge and watch the screen through the crack in the hinge side of the door. She was furious with Rod and me if we laughed.

Life was hectic, but I loved having lots of children around me. All the same, I was as relieved as any modern mum when bedtime came around and they became as near to angelic as they were likely to get! Delicate eyelids, long lashes resting on soft, smooth cheeks, soft breathing as they dreamt peacefully. Could that be the boy who hated me this morning and was sorry this afternoon . . . could this be the small girl who had screamed that she was never going to speak to me again - that is, until after her bath when I got a great big wet hug? The few years I spent at home with my children before I returned to work were certainly among my happiest, and at times, some of my most frustrating. Bringing up children has never been easy, but I think it must be extremely difficult in today's world where there is so much more influence from outside the home and school.

I was lucky that the children's three grandparents took them out whenever they could but my husband rarely came with us because of his marshalling activities for the motor race meetings. Sometimes I felt quite rebellious about the fact that other parents took their children out together at the weekends or they were able to stay with family or friends, or even take a holiday when there was a Bank Holiday. We could never do that because race meetings were always held at such times. In later years, however, when we were both retired and mostly together for 24 hours a day, I came to enjoy the days when Rod was away and I could do what I wished!

CHAPTER FIFTEEN

HOLIDAYS, GOOD AND BAD

For today's youth, the world, it seems, has become their oyster. Back in the 1960s, the idea of foreign travel was something that few ordinary people could afford. The contrast between holiday aspirations then and now is stark. When Lee was three and Krista one, we managed a week in a holiday camp at Littlestone-on-Sea, a small coastal village near New Romney in Kent. Holiday camps were very popular, providing entertainment and amusement for adults and children in all weathers. This was a big advantage over staying in a boarding house, where we were unwelcome indoors after breakfast.

Our chalet accommodation at the camp was little more than wooden shed raised slightly above the ground with a small veranda. The beds were iron- framed, with doubles always appearing to sag into the middle. A small chest was provided, but the drawers always stuck - presumably the winter damp got to them. There was a single wardrobe and a wash basin. Sanitation was an enamel chamber pot and a slop bucket, which had to be carried across the greens in front of the chalets to a toilet block for emptying each morning. These chamber pots were often seen on the gables of the chalets occupied by young single men and women in the morning after their nightly partying.

Of this first holiday with Lee and Krista, I recall one incident in particular. Children could have an early tea, then be put to bed while parents had their evening dinner. Chalet maids patrolled the chalets and any crying was reported to the parents over the tannoy. My dinner was interrupted by a request for me to return to the chalet at once. Rod and I rushed out wondering what on earth had happened as we had left our children fast asleep and they did not normally wake up unless they were ill or disturbed. The walk from the dining room was some distance across a green and as we ran out I saw people stopping as they went past our chalet and then walking on laughing. I could see my small son's face at the open window and as we drew nearer I could hear the words that were making everyone laugh.

Complete with his pyjama trousers down around his ankles, my red-faced little boy was shouting for all the world to hear: 'Mummy! I have done a big bit in the potty, but I can't find the paper to wipe my bottom! MUMMEEEE!! Come quick!' Amazingly, his sister remained asleep through his pronouncements!

Our next holiday was one we had not really planned as money was so tight. We had had no holiday for about five years when my parents heard of a caravan through a friend of a friend. It was in a field in Dymchurch, another Kent village, and belonged to an elderly lady. It was quite cheap, so we saved up to take the children for one week. On the Saturday we arrived, the weather was not too bad. Wonderful, we thought - fresh air, the sea not too far away with a sandy beach, plenty of grass for the children to play and perhaps they would make new friends. Alas, the illusion was shattered almost as soon as we reached the caravan. It was just a few feet from a field where sheep grazed and from where there was an awful smell. We suspect this was caused by muck spreading. Inside the caravan, everything was dirty - especially all the cooking utensils. They were blackened and caked with food and the meat tin contained a solidified inch of cooking fat. Beneath the mattresses were jam sandwiches and melted fruit pastilles.

There was no electricity, no sanitation and both lighting and cooking were by camping gas. It was clear my first day would be spent in cleaning, but as I was determined the children would have a holiday Rod and I told them to play outside while we scrubbed the place and produced some sort of order from the chaos. I was relieved that at least we had our own, clean bedding.

The children soon informed me that they had made a friend, a little girl staying in the next caravan with just her mother. Good, I thought, that will be nice for them. It was - but not for Rod and me, as it turned out. The mother was a neurotic scrounger whose husband (quite justifiably in our view) had left her. She attached herself to us like a limpet for the rest of the week, constantly saying: 'You don't mind if I join you, do you.' It was not a question but rather a statement, until we finally said that we were going to see someone for the day and she could not come with us. It was such a relief not to have her constantly complaining about her husband.

That holiday was also memorable in other ways. On the second day we went in the sea and I hung my swimsuit on the line outside the caravan. The next morning it had gone! I could not afford another one, but it mattered little as we wore our raincoats for the rest of the holiday. I got a urinary infection and had to cross the field in the pitch dark and rain several times a night for the toilet. I spent a day at the local hospital when the infection became more serious, needing immediate treatment.

Mercifully, there were lighter moments. At breakfast one morning, Krista suddenly asked: 'Mummy, if you died and Daddy got married again, what would I be to the new Mummy?' What had made her ask that? Was my husband being unfaithful? Had the limpet in the next caravan said something untoward to Krista? Stay calm, I thought, just answer the question honestly.

'Well, dear,' I ventured, 'you would be her stepdaughter.'

But Krista countered: 'No! I meant would I be a bridesmaid?' It had always been her heart's desire to be one and it seems she thought the only way of achieving this was to get her father to marry someone else! I thought I must try harder to understand her questions before jumping to conclusions.

The holiday ended with another mini-drama – and with Rod and me vowing never to take another caravan break. As we were making our bed, he made to kiss me, saying how sorry he was that our holiday had been 'so disastrous.' I raised my arm – only to catch the lighted gas mantle, which fell down onto the blankets and set them alight. So the week that began with me having to clean up seemingly everything in sight ended with frantic efforts to douse our blazing bedclothes!

Once both our children had settled into school life, I began to think I could pursue some of my own interests and maybe find a job. I was not particularly well qualified; I had become the archetypal housewife and mother. And who in the world of business, I pondered, was looking for such a person, let alone one with a paralysed arm? I soon found that the part-time job I sought was not going to fall into my lap. I wanted to do more than just keep house, shop and cook. I felt evening classes might help and so, having been to Art College, I made a start at an oil painting class at an adult education centre – with a surprise outcome.

Sometime after joining the class I changed direction. 'This girl gives me lots of ideas,' said the man who was painting a picture in front of me, for by then I was no longer a student, I could not turn a hair, or blink, or change my expression - I had become an artist's model! I had soon discovered that my class needed costume models. Models were paid by the local education authority at an hourly rate. I thought this would be ideal for me - some pin money, an outside interest, meeting people whose lives were not necessarily dominated by home and family. I volunteered and was readily accepted – but any preconceptions about myself were soon shattered. As one woman said: 'It's so nice to have someone to pose who is not too good-looking; someone motherly.' I had not pictured myself like that at all! Then I discovered from the students' comments that my nose is on one side of my face, my skin is green, one eye is larger than the other, and my hair changed colour from week to week. I heard one man tell the tutor: 'Her hair is much redder this week.'

'Yes,' said the tutor, 'I expect she's tinted it!' Cue inward indignation as I had not even given it a coloured rinse for two years. Another man was rather annoyed as I had changed the colour of my lipstick from the previous sitting and he felt he ought to paint my lips again. I began to realise that for most of the students an artist's model was not a human being with ears to hear and eyes to see, but a solid mass to be interpreted according to their views or fantasies. Perhaps that is the difference between amateurs and professionals - the ability to interpret the inner personality of the sitter as well as the outer shell.

Sometimes when I entered the class, I felt as if I was walking through a hall of distorted mirrors, as I viewed the various manifestations of me. My hair was painted any colour from white to bright purple; it was actually dark brown at the time. I eventually took on more sessions working evenings and afternoons for two to two-and-a-half hours. I usually sat for about 20 minutes and then had a short break. Each class took about three sessions to complete their painting, although a few took six weeks.

The first time I sat, I fell asleep because the room was so hot. Next thing I knew, the tutor was gently shaking my shoulder and saying: 'I'm afraid you have slipped sideways in your sleep!' I lifted a very red face to look at a circle of grins! I thought it was the end of my new venture, but it made no difference. I sat for a number of other tutors after that - and always kept awake. I so enjoyed the evenings that a few pins and needles or even an aching muscle were worth it. I often felt quite invisible as a person, so I could observe those around me, mentally sort out problems or just plan next week's menus in my head. Some 30 years later, I met someone whose face I knew but could not place. 'I've got the most dreadful painting of you at home!' she said. 'You sat for the class I was in and when I took the painting home and showed my husband he said he hoped I would never show it to the poor woman as it was likely she would be most offended.'

CHAPTER 16

ILLNESS, FLOODS – AND LETTERS

Life, it seemed, was rarely dull – still less so when Rod was suddenly taken ill. It began in March, 1968, when he became unwell in the night. This was doubly shocking as he had rarely suffered anything more than a cold since his childhood polio, and he was never off sick. Now he had stomach pains; as we had been out the previous evening, I first thought something he had eaten had disagreed with him. I gave him Milk of Magnesia to drink, hopefully to settle his stomach – only to learn later that this could have killed him! The pains got worse; he was sick and began to turn green. I ran to the nearest phone box to call the doctor, who was soon with us. He suspected appendicitis with his appendix about to burst. A nurse later told me the medicine I had given him could well have precipitated the burst and possibly peritonitis. Rod was rushed to hospital, but I could not go with him because our children were still sleeping. My neighbours were too elderly to be knocked up at such an early hour, so I had to wait to find out what was happening to him.

Rod was operated on before lunch that day and – when they were not at work - my parents came to help with the children so that I could visit him. Rod's mother was staying with his brother and her little mongrel dog Squib was living with us while she was away. He was a great comfort, but now I wished more than ever that we had a phone in the house. Instead, we had a sort of grapevine network to pass on news. I would ring my parents at a specific time with a bulletin on Rod's health. His mother would ring my parents one hour later from a phone box about one mile from where she was staying, to hear how her son was getting on.

Few of us today consider what effect the telephone, especially mobiles has had on our lives, but if we consider how much we use it and from where, how things would be if we could only communicate in other ways, then we might appreciate more its impact on our lives. Computer technology and the Internet could have advanced little without the technology, which came from telecommunications. Letter-writing was still my most common means of communicating with friends and family.

My husband went into his company's convalescent home in Bournemouth before he resumed work after his operation. I was able to go and stay at a hotel for one night before visiting him. This is an extract from my letter to an Aunt.

24th April 1968

. . . . . I had a lovely bedroom with a toilet & telephone, Rod rang just as I got there and again at about 8.30a.m. I had a pot of tea & my newspaper brought up to my room then I went down to breakfast, you should have seen me, - my own table with my own silver coffee service - fruit juice - huge piece of haddock - brown bread - marmalade etc. (Bit of a come down today eating a bowl of corn flakes standing up getting the kids breakfast!.

As you can see, I was not very sophisticated and had very rarely had the chance to stay in a hotel with star rating of any sort. I thought this to be the way very rich people lived. I was missing my husband very much and finding the children a handful. Here is part of an undated letter to my in-laws while Rod was still convalescing:

...... I am counting the hours until Rod comes home, cleaning and polishing like mad as I want everything nice for his return. I think Lee misses him, too, because he seems to have been extra-difficult in the last few days and has been having mad fits of rushing around yelling at the top of his voice. Last night he threw talcum powder all over the bathroom, absolutely everything was covered and - wow - it didn't 'arf pong. Then he got an eyelash in his eye and yelled "f... (four letter word) My eye!" So I had to give him a good talking to this morning and today he has been a bit better. They went back to school last Wednesday much to the relief of Mums and residents alike. ....

My weight has always been a problem and was reflected in the following letter. We had been invited to a cousin's wedding.

5 September 1968

..... On Tuesday (my) Mum and I went to Lewisham as Mum wanted to get herself something for the wedding and insisted on getting me something; she was so sure C&A would have plenty for me, I was equally sure they wouldn't and I was right. You would think I was a freak monster because I don't want to dress as if I'd escaped from the ark. I had quite made up my mind to wear what I already had, but Mum kept on going from shop to shop until the children and my tempers were completely frayed, so in the end I said 'yes' so am busy chopping six inches off the bottom of a crimplene dress and coat that I don't really need for a wedding I don't particularly want to go to!....

When the day of the wedding dawned, it was raining hard but I dressed the children in their new finery and I donned the hated crimplene dress and coat. My father and mother collected the three of us for our drive to the church. As the ceremony began, I could hear a tremendous storm starting outside. The sky was rent by lightning, thunder crashed and boomed, echoing around the church and darkening the sky. It was like night. The rain was so heavy it began to drip through the roof, spattering guests and pews. The ceremony was catholic and very long. The children began to fidget; they were distracted by the storm. It became difficult to hear the priest conducting the ceremony, but Lee noticed he was sipping from a silver chalice from time to time. 'What is he doing Mummy?' came in a stage whisper from Lee. 'He is sipping the wine,' I said, and for a short while this satisfied him, but he watched the priest dip down behind the altar after the chalice had again been sipped. Suddenly, during a lull in the cacophony outside, his voice rang out: 'If he drinks any more of that wine, he will be stoned out of his mind!!' My acute embarrassment was only slightly mollified by the stifled laughter in the pew behind.

The rains did not subside and a few days after this Dartford was hit by floods. I was out shopping at the time, with the little dog Squib. I heard shoppers say the River Darent was rising; I thought perhaps I had better get out of the town as it is so low lying in the valley between two hills. I did not expect the flood to come so quickly; as I walked back through the town, the roads began to turn into rivers and lakes. I had to pass my husband's club, Acacia Hall, at the edge of the town, where it was once an old mill bridging the river; this was the point of entry for the water now rushing through the streets. It suddenly gushed out in a big wave as I reached the gates and I had to grab the dog under my good arm and hold the shopping up in order to wade through and up the hill on the other side. The dog was terrified and I feared I would not stay on my feet, but I managed to get across in seconds.

The floodwater was around for several days, but I had run out of fresh food. So when the water had receded from part of the town, I walked there to get what I could. I could not go by the most direct route, which was about a mile, so had to take an extra half-mile detour to the Co-op, where there was some food on the top shelves. I suppose the bottom shelves were still drying out. It was not very easy wading back through the town with my Wellingtons in my shopping bag held high to prevent the water filling them. My bare feet seemed to find all the rubbish that had collected beneath the water level.

CHAPTER 17

BACK TO WORK & OUR FIRST CAR

It was increasingly difficult to make ends meet. As Christmas, 1968, approached, I looked harder for work – with "eventful," not to say shattering, results! I saw an advert for a temporary part-time shop assistant at the local Co-op store for the six-week period up until Christmas, from 11:00 am to 4:00 pm, to cover all the break periods. I was thrilled when I got the job.

On my first day, I was placed on the fancy goods counter. Big mistake! Among these fancy goods, were two weird-looking "birds," serenely dipping long necks into a glass of water. As each bird alternately dipped, children stopped to watch. The hope was that Mum would also stop and be encouraged to buy something. With a broad smile, I turned on the charm as my first customer approached. 'Good morning Madam, can I help you?'

No, she didn't want the dipping birds, but she did make a purchase. I almost jumped for joy at my first sale. But my joy was short-lived. As I handed her the change, I must have caught the birds - which literally went flying straight across the counter, fast followed by the glass of water, which crashed into a display of glass swans. Moments earlier, the swans had been reposing on a glass mirror representing a lake.

The peace was well and truly shattered! Pity the lake wasn't real - I might have been able to persuade the customer they were diving ducks! At least, those of the swans remaining in one piece were now swimming in real water. At least, the mirror did not break. But the noise had attracted the attention of my new supervisor, a long suffering lady (or at least she was while I worked there). With a pained look, as she helped me mop up all the water and broken glass, she said: 'Never mind, dear, I expect it is first day nerves!'

I feared this would be my first and last day here, but the wages were so low that I think they were prepared to tolerate a clumsy idiot for a bit longer. Sometime later, I was transferred to travel goods. Whoops! Second big mistake. Selling handbags, purses and shopping trolleys presented few problems and nor did suitcases, provided people carried them away without wrapping. The day came when a customer wanted a large suitcase completely wrapped. Maybe you have never tried wrapping a large parcel mainly using one hand, but it was definitely not one of my strong points. I produced brown paper and sticky tape, both of which seemed to have a life of their own and which certainly did not harmonise with mine. The sticky tape attached itself first to me, then to the display stand and finally to the brown paper, only not in the right place. The brown paper crumpled, tore and ended up on the floor - three times. The embarrassed customer at last said 'Can I give you a hand, Miss?'

'How kind,' I said as he placed a tentative finger on the fourth sheet, which I promptly stuck down with the sticky tape. I think at this point he realised discretion was the better part of valour and said he would be happy to take the parcel as it was. He paid and promptly left the shop, trailing a fast disintegrating parcel. I wonder if he ever returned.

Just before Christmas I was put back on china and glass. That was the manager's third mistake. Some people never learn. Fortunately, the dipping ducks had flown the nest, or perhaps they had all been sold, so I thought I was fairly safe. The swans were still there, though, filled with pretty coloured water on their mirror lake. They were sold empty in a box with small pieces of variously coloured crepe paper, which the customer was supposed to soak in a jug of water to bring out the colour. This was then poured into the swan via the tail. There was no stopper.

I was approached by a customer who wanted to buy a swan from the display with coloured water already inside. I explained they could not be sold with the water in because there were no stoppers and the glass from which they were made was thin and fragile, so they were carefully packed in boxes. But the customer insisted: 'I want one from the display.' I patiently explained again, in more detail.

by Barbara Blackston Huntley

'I WANT ONE FROM THE DISPLAY, A BLUE ONE!' shouted the customer.

'Just a moment, Madam, I will get the supervisor,' I replied, not believing that someone was prepared to carry home a very fragile swan that might shatter, covering them with blue dye (many had been returned by customers who found them broken in the box by the time they had reached home).

The supervisor duly repeated my explanation. 'GET ME THE MANAGER!' stormed the irate customer. I got the manager telling him what had already occurred. He smiled at the customer and said: 'If Madam wishes to have a display swan, we can certainly sell it to her.'

I passed Madam a swan containing blue water.

'I want it wrapped,'

'But Madam,' I began to stutter, 'the water will run out into the box'.

'I have to go home on the bus and I WANT IT WRAPPED!'

I stood the box on its side and very gently put the swan inside. I placed the whole in a bag, hoping Madam would make it to the bus stop before the blue dye trickled from the box. My colleagues and I fell about laughing when the poor woman had finally left; we all pictured a widening blue stain spreading over the passengers in the bus.

My last day, Christmas Eve, was almost as eventful as the first. I was to work until the shop closed at 5.30 pm. Soon after 4:00 pm, drunken men began to pour into the shop to buy last-minute presents for their wives or girlfriends. They shouted and jockeyed for position near the counter, calling 'Miss, Miss, me next.' I was desperately running up and down the counter trying to serve everyone as quickly as I could. There were no tills for the cash, just a lockable drawer with a board inside with round holes cut in it. Each hole had a wooden bowl inside in which the different coins were kept. My feet ached, my head ached and I desperately wanted the afternoon to end. As I rushed to give a particularly loud customer his change, I pulled out the change drawer with some force. It shot right out of the counter, clattering to the floor and scattering change everywhere. Coins ran under the counter and into all the nooks and crannies. A great shout went up from the merry customers, who all offered at once to help to pick it up. I just thought 'thank God it's my last day.' To my great surprise, I received a letter thanking me for my valued contribution and saying I was welcome to return at any time. I take it the letter was a work of fiction - either that or the Co-op should beware of sending standard letters!

Being a devil for punishment, I then found a job in a greengrocers. I was a bit more at home among the potatoes and cabbages, but even here life had its moments. An old man came in with a home-made wooden wheelbarrow and wanting to buy a cabbage on a top shelf. As I reached up, he went forward to point out his choice, but in so doing pushed the wheelbarrow into the back of my knees. My knees promptly folded, sending me backwards into his barrow! My colleagues couldn't hide their amusement as they helped free me from the box-like contraption in which I was now firmly wedged. The bruises were more to my pride than my body.

Bruising of a different kind came with an incident in the rear of the shop, where I had gone to replenish some stock. Each day the owner of a local cafe would call to collect salad vegetables. Now I was suddenly aware of him approaching me with a box of tomatoes held on his head with one arm. His other arm shot out and grabbed me around the waist. His face came down on mine and he kissed me hard on the lips. My rubber-gloved good hand whacked him really hard across his face and the tray of tomatoes crashed to the floor. I escaped his clumsy clutches and rushed back into the shop. A few moments later he passed through with red marks along his cheek, but without comment. He continued to come into the shop, but neither of us ever mentioned the incident again - although he always had a wary eye when he passed me.

Then there was the tale of the tiny potatoes. The woman in charge was always keen to get rid of sub-standard produce, either before displaying new stock or mixing the "subs" with the new. Men, seen as less discerning shoppers, were usually easy targets. I had wanted to put out a new bag of potatoes, as there were only very tiny chats left in the bin, but I was told I must sell these first. A man bought 12 lbs (approx. 5.5 kilos) of these tiny potatoes - he looked a bit surprised but said nothing. About one hour later, his enraged wife stormed into to the shop. 'What on earth do you mean by selling my husband these?' she fumed. 'You can have them back!' With that, she promptly upturned the bag and emptied the lot all over the floor, causing quite a rumpus among our startled customers. Soon after this incident, I found a job even closer to home in a little general store. Strangely enough, the short while I worked there passed without too many problems - but I think I had already realised retailing was not for me. Two goods arms are a definite advantage for shop work!

In April, 1969, my father retired after 46 years with the GPO (General Post Office). He bowed out as a Leading Technical Officer in charge of Crayford Telephone Exchange. He was 60 and in poor health, the result of never fully recovering from the ankylosing spondylitis and stomach ulcers he had suffered when he was 25, and also the lack of the correct diet with wartime rationing. He was quite relieved to be able to leave five years before normal retirement age, but it meant he had to live for five years on the £2,000 gratuity which was his reward for 46 years of loyal service. He also received the Queen's medal for long service, presented to him by the Manager at the telephone exchange. He had a small pension, but there was no provision for my mother in the event of his death.

I attended the retirement ceremony, with Mum, and we heard all about his 24-hour vigils during the war, when it was essential to keep telephone lines repaired after air raid bombing in the London exchanges where he was working. As well as his normal duties, he did all the cooking for the engineers who were working through the night. All telephone exchanges were manually run at that time so there was a large labour force. Fine words are often soon forgotten by the people who say them, but with the passing of the years I realise that the reward of service to others is the value it gives to one's self - the satisfaction of striving to meet the standard we have set for ourselves. Maybe that sounds pompous, but we can only ever really achieve our own goals. I always admired what my father achieved despite the real hardships in those times and his tenacity and hard work in the face of many health problems.

Rod, meanwhile, desperately wanted to learn to drive. He wanted lessons - to see if he would make a capable driver - before buying a car. This seemed an impossible dream as no-one in the area had a car adapted with hand controls suitable for him to drive with his polio-paralysed leg. The Ministry of Health provided Minis for the severely disabled, so Rod wrote to the Ministry, explaining his problem. However, they said he could only have help if he was totally handicapped. He explained that he was not seeking financial help; he just wanted a hand-controlled vehicle for lessons before borrowing the money for a car he might not be able to drive. They suggested he write to the AA, but they could not help, either.

For five years, he sought someone who could provide an adapted car. He even contacted our local MP and BSM (British School of Motoring), who were said to have facilities for the disabled, but still to no avail. We phoned the BSM's head office and they told us they had a suitable car in another town about four miles away. Alas, it transpired that this car, with hand controls, had recently been disposed of, and so there was no help here.

By now, we were virtually resigned to struggling forever, getting on and off buses weighed down with all our shopping and two children in tow. Then a chance meeting with Mr Haskins, a local driving instructor who owned his own school gave us the breakthrough. Mr Haskins wanted to help, but could not at first see how. A week later, he had a solution. He bought a new car for his driving school and said he was prepared to fit hand controls to the new vehicle if Rod would buy them from him when he passed his driving test. Rod was delighted and in March, 1969, he had his first lesson. He passed his driving test first time nine months later. It was the best possible Christmas present. Then we secured a bank loan and bought our first second-hand car.

CHAPTER 18

ADAPTING TO NEW JOBS . . . AND CHANGING TRENDS

While my father was settling down to retirement, I was seeking pastures new in the employment world – and this time ended up working for the same company as Rod. I was interviewed for a full-time job as a stock records clerk with The Wellcome Foundation (formerly Burroughs Wellcome & Co.). I was quite nervous about this interview as it was with a very reputable organisation. My real concern was that I could not hold out my right hand when meeting someone for the first time; if I held out my left hand, the other person became confused and embarrassed. My application stated that I had polio in my right arm. So the foxy-faced interviewer – having been forewarned, I guess - offered neither hand on introduction. I hoped he would forgive me for not shaking hands. In the event, he was more concerned about my polio arm than my academic ability or experience.

'How will you manage with your disability?' he asked, eyeing my arm uncertainly.

'I don't know how I will cope with this particular job,' I replied. 'I can only say I have no difficulty with writing; I have brought up two children, been an embroidery designer and served in shops without any major problems. My only difficulty is lifting heavy weights from above my head.' (I didn't say: 'Apart, that is, from dipping ducks, large suitcases and drawers without backstops.') He asked hardly anything about my qualifications for the job, which was just as well, really, because I had so few.

'Well, Mrs Blackston,' he declared, 'I am prepared to give you a three-month trial if the head on the packing materials section agrees. I will of course have to talk to him first and you will have to take a test.' For good measure, Mr Foxy-Face added pompously: 'If we feel the job is not suitable for you with your disability, then of course we must protect ourselves and you would not be allowed to continue.'

I passed their mathematical test and was given a date to start work in May, 1969. On my first morning, I reported to Personnel and was taken to my new office along an internal factory road bordered by high black buildings. The one I was to work in had been an old mill and stood at the edge of a large mill pond fed by the River Darent. At one end of the building was an iron fire escape and I had to climb this to reach my new office.

I was to work in the Packaging Materials Section of Production Control for £11 a week. The job involved manually calculating quantities of packing materials required to pack drugs from a works order, then entering on card the stocks required and how much remained available. At that time the only machinery in the offices were adding machines, large cumbersome objects. There were no calculators and certainly no computers. The stock mostly comprised bottles for tablets, creams or liquid medicines, cartons, foil for tablets, vials for injections and labels. The works orders came in each day, saying how much of a drug was to be packed (number of tablets, bottles of medicine, quantity of vaccine etc.). Each clerk had to calculate mentally, or on rough paper, how much or how many of the appropriate packing materials would be needed for a specific number of products to be packed.

I found the most difficult calculations were for tin foil. It was always calculated by weight per number of products, for example: 1 lb. of foil would pack a million tablets. If the works order said the packing run was to be 10,250 tablets we were expected to calculate the exact weight of foil needed for that run plus a small margin for errors. Too much would mean the price of the finished pack was too high and profit was lost; too little for the drug taken out of stock for packing might have meant the drug had to be destroyed, again destroying profit. This was crucial with vaccines as their shelf life and storage conditions were very limited. Labels had to be printed with batch numbers and expiry dates as well as product information. So great care in the allocation of stock was important because these items could not be returned to stock once printed.

My section head was Mr Summers, a Christian Scientist man with a religion-based strict code of behaviour, but he was very fair. I was also very grateful to him later on when he 'saved my bacon.' I liked my new job and soon picked up the work. Two other clerks had started just a month earlier and we were a lively group, generally getting on fairly well together. There was just one lady who was eternally miserable; she saw only the bad side of everything and for the rest of us it was a challenge to get a good word or cheerful remark out of her. A good example was my own feeble effort one sunny spring day, when the birds were singing and the whole world seemed wonderful. 'What a lovely day!' I said, convinced that Mrs Misery could not fault such an innocent comment. 'It's far too good to be at work!' she retorted venomously. I did not try too much after that to cheer her up.

A few months into the job, I had to calculate the packing materials for a very large run of polio vaccine. I made a dreadful error by omitting a nought from the quantity of materials to be used. A large quantity of very expensive vaccine had to be destroyed and a packing run aborted. My section head explained the awful consequences and I felt the most dreadful shame; I was doubly appalled for the fact that polio vaccine had been involved. My section head was obviously very worried, but he tried to reassure me whilst making me realise the enormity of what I had done. I later discovered that he took the blame for the incident himself and would not tell his superiors which clerk had made the error. Instead, he said he was the person responsible for the clerk's work and he took the blame. He did not tell me this and of course I had feared I would lose my job. When I found out what he had done, I was overwhelmed to think that someone could be so courageous. My admiration for him was boundless. I decided there and then that if ever I was in a senior position, and someone made a genuine mistake, I would try to emulate this man. When later promotions came my way, I always remembered the way he did things and tried to model myself on him, although I did not always succeed.

Section heads were all male, as were most supervisors; they were all addressed as 'Mr.' A few senior clerks were women; they and all the clerks were addressed by their first names.

Women were paid much less than men and were very much second class; they were not expected to wear trousers at any time, regardless of the weather. I once went to work in trousers when the weather was absolutely freezing and there was frost on the inside of the windows; it caused quite a sensation as nobody had dared to wear them in the office before. I was called into the senior manager's office and asked if I was trying to start a new fashion. I said I was just trying to keep warm - but was firmly told trousers were not acceptable wear for a woman under any circumstances! The poor manager almost had apoplexy when in the summer the fashion for hot pants came in and two of the young, more rebellious, long- legged girls came in wearing very short ones in bright colours. They were sent home to change immediately.

My trousers incident was in early 1971, when the miners went on strike. This resulted in lengthy power cuts, day and night, and even led to a three-day working week for many. We carried on in our office when we could, going in early or staying later according to when power was available or when there was enough daylight. I wonder what would happen now if there were such long periods of time without power, when we are so utterly dependent on electricity for computers to run everything. It might yet happen, of course. In 1971, shops and offices were able to carry on and our main worry at home was whether we could have a hot meal on return from work.

The firm's social club at Acacia Hall was very popular with all the employees, at lunch times and evenings. Rod and I, with some colleagues, soon formed a group that regularly went to dances there. I felt very well off now that I could earn my own money and was thoroughly enjoying my new- found freedom. However, £3 of my £11 wages had to pay someone to care for my children after school and to help do some housework and ironing. My parents had more freedom since Dad's retirement. They often helped with little jobs around the house and would take the children out on picnics and to the various parks in the area. Greenwich Park was a big favourite; they spent many happy hours there.

My father enjoyed driving then, when there was far less traffic than now and the countryside was easily accessible, with plenty of places for picnicking or just strolling about. With very few motorways, people were not so inclined to drive from A to B as fast as possible. They could pause by the roadside with a flask of tea or coffee, set up a little table and chairs and watch the traffic go by as they refreshed themselves.

We both seemed to cope reasonably well with our children and jobs, although at times I got quite exhausted. When I read old diaries, I realise we must have had a lot of energy to combine full-time work, dashing to and fro with the children to our parents, guides or scouts, decorating the house, visiting or entertaining friends and relatives, and going to parties. Rod also served on the parents and supporters committee of the scouts, helping with fund raising etc. as well as his weekend trips to Brand's Hatch to marshal at the motor racing. My weekends were taken up with shopping, washing and almost every week I made batches of cakes or pies. The shops did not open late in the evenings or Sundays, so Saturday was a mad rush day for me.

This is a letter I wrote to a local newspaper in 1973, when I had been with the company for four years. I think it rather summed up my attitude. It was in reply to someone who thought all firms should have crèches for children. This was a revolutionary idea at the time - but the era of women's liberation was just beginning.

Dear Sirs,

I was keenly interested in "KT Talking point" (July 20). Mrs Hunter has a very valid argument for crèche facilities within industry but I don't think employers will go to the considerable expense of providing them.

Many mothers of very young children tend to be unreliable in their attitude to work, naturally their children come first. A mother with a young child will have to cope with bouts of chickenpox, mumps, measles, coughs, etc. In early schooldays there are sports days and medicals to attend and a mother must decide whether to support her child or her employer.

A mother's job may be exhausting mentally but woe-betide her if she comes home too tired to listen to her children's troubles. She must cook, shop and do the housework in the evenings, lunch hours and weekends, plus making sure the children get their outings at the weekends.

She will probably wrestle with a guilty conscience about who comes first and when. She must also remember her husband, he may be, as mine is, a wonderful support and help but he too comes home tired. Nobody is at their best every day. Both husband and wives may come home with problems but they must prepare meals, bath the children then catch up on household jobs before sitting down, and though they may well have plenty of interesting things to say to each other the temptation may be just to sit in front of the television.

An employer knows these things and is wary of married women with young children.

I am very much in favour of married women with children having the opportunity to work, but they must realise what they are letting themselves in for and remember employers are not charitable institutions.

I am a working mother who has been in full-time employment for the last four years, my youngest child was seven years when I began and I paid about a quarter of my wages to get help with the house work. I no longer have this help and of course my children are much more independent now. I have had wonderful support during past school holidays from both my parents and my mother-in-law, and am blessed with two very healthy children. I enjoy working.

Going to work certainly eases the financial burden on a family but time must be found to enjoy the extra cash.

Admittedly I feel more of a person in my own right now and not just "the other half," but it would be wrong to say it is all marvellous, I have had many a battle with my conscience and sometimes I've thought I could not cope but it has always worked out in the end. However I don't think many mothers can cope without support.

Some do not have a husband and sadly they are forced into a situation, but for those who do have the choice I would say think carefully how you will manage.

To me the support of my family has been essential, a crèche would have been useful but not the complete answer to the problem.

Yours faithfully...'

I wrote this letter when there were far fewer single parents than now and most children were born to married couples. Things were starting to change; it was the era of 'flower power' and so-called 'free love,' but none of this touched me. I just read about it in the newspapers. I wonder if the letter still has relevance to today's couples or whether the changes in society mean that women feel guilty if they do not go to work.

I must have been reasonably successful in the eyes of my superiors because after one year I was promoted to senior clerk and also elected as the staff representative on the company's Junior Staff Consultative committee. This was a toothless committee for the airing of staff views on wages and working conditions and was supposed to help with management decision-making. I became known as a rebel because I was never happy being a 'yes' woman. I sometimes gave the management team rather an uncomfortable ride. It probably had little effect, but at least we were eventually allowed to wear trouser suits - but definitely not slacks! I managed to get more lighting in our dark offices and also learnt of pay rises about 20 minutes before other staff!

My original section head was promoted and moved to another area. I missed him for his fairness and understanding, but his religion forbade him from celebrating Christmas. Our new boss was somewhat younger; he was not a bad boss, but we did not have quite the same respect for him.

I, on the other hand, was a rather strict senior clerk. I would not tolerate lateness and tended to stick to the rules fairly rigidly. This made me unpopular at times, but as I had always been a bit of a loner I was not worried by this. Lack of respect, though, was something else. I hope over the years I learned some wisdom and tolerance, but it was a long time coming. Sticking to the rule book rebounded on me some years later in another job, but it did teach me a lesson I never forgot. Bending the rules is part of human nature and as long as the bending is petty then it is probably a good idea to accept it in order to enforce the rules that really matter for the safety and well-being of all.

My job altered somewhat over time and I became a stock auditor, checking that the stock recorded matched that held in the stores. If there was a discrepancy, this had to be traced if at all possible. I enjoyed this as it was often detective work in the sense that there were various reasons for such discrepancies. Sometimes it was put in the wrong place, sometimes it was recorded incorrectly or sometimes it was stolen.

In my last year with the company – 1974 - I was moved to another section after a number of operations on my arm (see next chapter). I was travelling to Crewe each month, forecasting stock requirements for the coming year. It was exhausting and for four months my paralysed arm was encased in a very heavy plaster. I usually stayed over one or two nights. As well as my overnight needs, I had to carry a very heavy briefcase containing printouts of music-ruled continuous computer paper. This was produced by a large central computer department isolated behind locked doors; other staff could make no direct input to these machines. Everything was recorded on special forms, then punched in by staff within that department.

My new section head immediately disliked me and I him. It was a big personality clash and led to me suddenly giving in my notice when I could no longer stand his arrogant attitude. My health was in a poor state because of my operations and I was depressed and upset.

I regretted my decision - without seeking another job first - because I desperately needed the money. I need not have worried, though. Before my one month's notice was finished, I had found new work. I had been with Wellcome for five-and-a-half years and left with many happy memories and very few unhappy ones except for my last year, 1974. My return to work whilst suffering the traumas left by my operations had left me severely depressed. I needed time to adjust to the way my arm now worked and I wanted far less responsibility. The new job was less money, but one I could do very easily. It was ideal for my situation at the time.

CHAPTER NINETEEN

HAPPINESS, HOPE AND FAILURE

My life changed the day I bought a new pair of shiny black plastic boots. It all started on a weekend away from the family, staying with an aunt in her flat in Holland Park. As I had saved a few pounds for the trip we decided on a shopping spree in South Kensington. I hunted for a pair of boots to fit my thin ankles and thick calves. It was January, 1973, and I had £10 to spend, but initially all boots were either too expensive or not my size. At last, I found a pair of stretchy plastic ones with clumpy soles and heels for £4.50 in a sale. I was so proud of these that I wore them home on Sunday. I had forgotten about the highly polished floor in my hallway - I slipped over and wrenched my knee. I picked myself up, hoped I hadn't done any damage, and forgot about it until the next day - when my knee was very painful and swollen. I went to work thinking it would eventually go away, but after six weeks of pain I decided to see the doctor who advised seeing a specialist.

I had to wait a long time for my appointment and in the meantime I had lost my long-serving cleaning lady. Sue was the sort of gem who is never fully appreciated until she leaves. She had worked for me six hours a week, allowing me to come home to a clean and tidy house. This was well worth the few pounds I paid her and let me devote weekends to the children and cooking and helping my now increasingly dependent mother-in-law.

My knee swelling began to go down and I thought about cancelling my hospital appointment. I decided to keep it as the knee still hurt. I told the consultant I felt a bit of a fraud, as it was much better. He said he thought it would heal itself in due course, but then he noticed my polio arm. He asked what had happened and what treatment I had received.

'If we could operate to improve it, how would you feel?' he said. My heart leapt! Could he really give me a second chance, the dream I had been waiting for, hoping that one day medical science could improve my paralysed arm? When my children were small, I had longed to hold them in both hands, to raise them above my head. I wished I could buy coats with cuffs at the wrist, but as the right one had always to be shortened by five inches (12cm) it was not practical. I longed to wear sleeveless dresses in public, but a thin, dislocated shoulder is not a pretty sight - so I generally avoided garments without sleeves. I wished I could pull up tights easily; I wished I could use both hands for my hideous 'roll-on' girdles. Sometimes, when I rushed into the loo and then tried to come out in a hurry, I would get in a terrible tangle with dresses or skirts tucked into knickers or girdle; people wondered what kept me so long. It was a great relief when corsets and girdles became part of history - I was glad to let it all hang out!

When I wore stockings, I had to be a contortionist to do the right back one up. I usually managed it, but pinging suspenders were an occupational hazard very familiar to me. Bras were okay. I have always found it fairly easy to do those up at the back with my left hand only, but the fashion for 'teddy' garments that did up under the crotch were quite beyond me. I bought one and managed to get it done up, but only after all sorts of bending and stretching over a bathroom stool. That was all right until I was at a dance with Rod and realised that my weak bladder could not withstand the pressure much longer. I just had to go, but there was the problem. The cubicle was designed for a size eight lady and I more than doubled that. Also, the toilet seat was unlikely to withstand the gymnastic display required for me to get the wretched 'teddy' done up. The top half was a lacy evening blouse which, when I could not do up the garment underneath, rode up above my waist to reveal a V-shaped piece of nylon back and front with pop-studs on the end! Although embarrassed, I saw the funny side, but I'm sure most of the other dancers saw it long before I did.

Shaving under arms was another hazardous job. Under the right arm, with my left hand, was no problem, but under the left arm – also with my left hand - was rather more difficult, although achievable. It seems awful to whinge about such small difficulties when people in wheelchairs face so many more trials, but I can't help thinking that shops and public places could give more thought to the problems of people with arm disabilities. It is not just people with paralysis or no arms, but also those who have arthritic hands and arms, not least the elderly. My pet hates are heavy doors, shopping trolleys which are difficult to manoeuvre with two hands, let alone one, and buffet meals where there is not an inch of space left to put a plate down in order to place food on it. Beware the single-handed person who drops prawns into the gateau whilst trying to balance a plate on the edge of two dishes or who falls headlong into the trifle while balancing on one leg, with the other raised to balance a plate on one knee!

Rant over, I return to my story of the consultant who had given me hope that one day I might be able to do the things that others did with ease. He said he would write to Donal Brooks, a surgeon at the Royal National Orthopaedic Hospital in Great Portland Street, London. If this man would see me, he was sure my arm could be greatly improved. I was to have a muscle test at my local hospital first, to see which muscles still operated and which were totally paralysed. This took place in June, 1973, when it was found that I used back muscles to move part of my upper arm, instead of the arm muscles normally used.

I was so excited when I left that hospital - I felt as people must do when they have won millions on the Lottery. I could not believe my luck in having a second chance. I was on cloud nine and so happy. I rushed home to tell everyone, bubbling over with the consultant's plans for me. The family were pleased for me, but not as enthusiastic as I was. They said I was brave to volunteer for non-essential surgery. I did not see it like that and nothing would have deterred me then or at any time prior to the first operation.

Maybe I would have been better prepared for the trauma that followed if I had listened to some of the warnings. Looking back, I suspect that much of what is thought 'brave' by others is actually an act of pure instinct; lack of forethought or love for another person can help an individual take a 'brave' action. For me, it was lack of forethought; I would never have accepted that my arm would not be better or could even be worse - although I was warned.

I got my appointment to see Mr Brooks in London. He thoroughly examined my arm and reviewed the muscle tests. These showed that there were no active muscles in the upper arm, none to hold the shoulder in the joint, and weak muscles in the lower arm, but there was a reasonable grip and some use of the fingers. The fingers were constantly curled up and could only be opened when the wrist was held rigid. The thumb muscles were paralysed and I could not use the thumb to touch my fingertips. My hand was almost back to front and could not be turned inwards. (I had learned some tricks with muscles in my upper back to move my shoulder and arm forward.)

Mr Brooks had suffered what I understood to be polio in his legs, so he had specialised in arm surgery, which he could mostly do in a sitting position. I liked him straightaway and felt I was in good hands. He suggested fixing my wrist into a rigid position with ulna bone cut from my lower forearm. This piece of bone, about two inches long, was to be cut up into small pieces and hammered into the wrist bones, which would eventually heal to form one bone from elbow to knuckles of the hand. This would give me more control of my fingers and allow them to open easily; it would also let my hand turn inwards. My arm would be in plaster for four months while the bones knitted together; it also meant that I would never be able to bend my wrist in any direction again.

The second stage was to be an operation to remove the strongest tendon from the middle finger and transfer it to my thumb in the hope that I would be able to pull it up. It was the least serious of the three operations and involved only a light back slab plaster for a few weeks. The third stage was to fuse my dislocated shoulder into the socket. This would give it a more normal profile and stop my arm hanging by the skin and ligaments; the deltoid muscle, which normally covers the shoulder, was paralysed, leaving my shoulder permanently hanging out of the socket. This also meant four months in plaster from waist to neck and down the arm. It could only be done in winter because heat could cause rashes under the plaster and sweating would make the whole thing very unpleasant. Once the operation was complete, it was unlikely I would ever be able to lie on my right side again. This was the stage that worried me most and the surgeon said he would try and introduce me to someone who had already had the operation.

I was given time to think things over. If I wished to proceed, I had to go before a panel of doctors and students who would assess my suitability, both mental and physical, for these operations. I had no doubt this was my chance to have a more useful right arm; I was prepared to go through anything to achieve that. I duly returned to meet the panel of doctors, including, I believe, a psychiatrist. I was full of enthusiasm, but it seemed the surgeon was trying to put me off. He said none of the operations was guaranteed to succeed. My chances of real improvement were 50/50; I might even be worse off and some of the procedures would be very uncomfortable. The whole thing would probably take between two and three years.

I remained adamant this was what I wanted. I was accepted and admitted to The Royal National Orthopaedic Hospital on November 11, 1973, just before my 36th birthday, for the first operation to fix my wrist. The orthopaedic ward was a lively one because many of the women there were not medically ill in themselves, but were recovering from orthopaedic operations. They often had to stay in hospital for long periods while bones were knitting, but they were otherwise reasonably well. One lady had been lying on her back for six weeks after a spinal operation.

The day of the operation, I was both nervous and excited; I knew it would take several hours. I had my pre-med and remember very little after that until the next day, when I came to in the recovery ward, where I was to spend the next 24 hours. A nurse at my bedside wet my dry lips when I asked for water. I could not believe the intensity of the pain now; it was excruciating, but as I moaned in agony I was given morphine. The next day, I was moved back to the ward and when I came to again my arm was strapped up above me, hanging from a stand in a type of sling. I could see four very fat, black sausages protruding from the plaster and bandages. They were unrecognisable as fingers. They grew fatter and were very black the next day and felt as if they would burst.

In the days that followed, I suffered nightmare dreams from hell, intense pain - and no escape route. My mother visited and said I had bitten through my lips, trying to stifle my tears, and they were bleeding. I was desperate that my children did not see me at this stage, with my courage gone. The children sent little notes and drawings, which meant so much to me. I felt very cowardly, not being able to hide my feelings; it taught me that it is easy to volunteer for what others may consider a brave action but the reality of going through with it is something else. I greatly admired others in the ward who had endured far worse than I had, especially the lady who had lain on her back for six weeks after a very traumatic spinal operation. She took her first steps while I was there, but it made her feel very nauseated. Another lady was brought into the ward having been unable to walk for 14 years; she had two hips replaced and walked out a few weeks later on sticks. They worked miracles in that hospital.

About three days after the operation, I had a strange experience when I was at rock bottom. I had told a woman on the ward that I was an atheist and so had no-one to believe in but myself and my own ability to recover from the unbearable pain - at the time, I just wanted to die. This woman said she was a catholic and found her religion a great comfort in dealing with her pain. The next morning her priest visited her and the curtains were drawn around her bed. I barely noticed what was going on, but shortly afterwards I began to feel much better; by the evening I was sitting up and laughing. I told the catholic lady: 'I have felt much better since about 11 o'clock this morning.' She said she and the priest had spent his visit praying for me and he had left about the time I had suddenly begun to feel better. I'm still an atheist, but I do sometimes feel that other people's faith can help you.

In spite of so much pain for so many, it was a very happy ward with an international team of dedicated nurses. Many of the patients, including me, liked a little tipple during recovery. Mine was martini; others had whisky and sloe gin. In the next bed to me an actress frequently had champagne delivered. It all helped provide a bit of party spirit.

A few weeks later, before I was due to leave hospital, I had to have my plaster changed under anaesthetic for the removal of stitches and wound cleaning. It was my birthday, but I could take nothing by mouth. When I came round, the patients had collected to buy me a birthday cake and some Chanel No. 5 perfume. I was very touched at such kindness and asked if I could have a piece of the cake. 'No!' said the nurse, 'you will be sick'. Eventually she gave in and I had a small piece - and was promptly sick. But it was worth it! Everyone had a piece and later that night we all had a little drink to celebrate, including some of the nurses. Not, though, the night staff, who came round with sleeping tablets later. For them it was a very peaceful night - and some of us were reluctant to wake up next morning!

I went home on November 28. I was delighted to be back with my family, but I remained severely restricted because my arm had to be kept raised above my head to allow fluids to drain away. The children welcomed me back, but then began to play up. It was as if they resented my being away from them and then all the attention I received on return. Lee was just 14 and Krista 12. I suppose it was hard for them to come to terms with what had happened to their normally active and well organised mother, who was now tearful and somewhat traumatised by the pain. I was full of bravado when visitors called, but very depressed at other times.

One memory stands out. I tried to resume my household duties as soon as I could. I began by cooking our evening meal, which Rod would prepare before work. One evening I put the oven on and lit the gas to cook the vegetables on top of the cooker. At that moment, Lee came home from school with the knee torn out of his trousers and a nasty wound underneath where he had fallen. (I suspect he may have been fighting). I stopped what I was doing to bathe his knee and when I finished I realised I had not put the dinner plates in the oven to warm up. My husband was due in at any moment, so I popped the plates on top of the simmering pans of vegetables.

Rod appeared and as he stood beside me at the cooker to put the kettle on there was a sudden explosion! The oven door flew open, sending a flame up the front of me and melting my clothes, which contained a lot of nylon. The side of Rod's trousers also melted. The wadding around the fingers of my plaster cast was singed, but I was not burned. I had put on the oven before Lee came in from school, but had not lit the gas. It had come up the oven flu at the back of the cooker and ignited from the gas rings on top, forcing the oven door open against me. In a way, it was fortunate that it was winter and I was wearing a number of layers, with only the top ones melting rather than flaming, but it was all very frightening.

After this, I was talking to the children about helping me when Krista said that it was my choice to have the operations and so she did not see why she should be given extra chores because of it. That really hurt, but she is older, wiser and kinder now. Lee always showed concern, but was rarely around when I needed his help. I suppose you could say he had a good bedside manner; he appeared to care a great deal, but his less willing sister ended up doing more chores - so I expect she felt that life was unfair. I never doubted my children's affections, but perhaps an organising mum who suddenly cannot cope is quite a shock to them, and maybe resentment can follow.

In the summer of 1974, I had a tendon transferred from the middle finger of my polio hand to the thumb. This was expected to allow my thumb to reach across to my fingers and perhaps allow me to pick things up more easily. Physiotherapy followed and I was told to move my middle finger; I tried, and my thumb rose slightly. My brain did not immediately know that the tendon was now connected to my thumb; however, after a few days, I was able to think 'thumb' rather than middle finger and it responded slightly. I was fascinated by the way messages were transferred from brain to hand and its ability to react to the changes made. Unfortunately, the tendon was left rather loose and the operation was not a success. It was redone in February, 1975, but although the tendon was shortened it was still not a success and could not be done again. I was very disappointed to say the least.

I think the failure of the last two operations, the mental strain of adjusting, depression about giving up my previous job and starting the new one led me to decide that I could not face the final operation on my right shoulder. I was very afraid it would go badly and that there could be no turning back. I chickened out and chose to leave things as they were.

So the dream was over. With hindsight, I was no better and no worse off than before. Some things were easier - like filing - and my hand now turned inwards, so was cosmetically better looking, although my right arm was still five inches shorter that my left. Sewing was now much harder, as was preparing vegetables, because my wrist could not bend. Using a knife was impossible for the same reason, but the hospital showed me a rocker knife shaped like a small axe which I could use to cut up meat with my left hand. I bought one and it has been really useful at home and I am still using it over 40 years later, but of course I don't have it when I eat out. I rarely order steak in a restaurant because it is so difficult to cut and it can be embarrassing to ask for it to be cut up in the kitchen as waiters/waitresses sometimes react and I feel I have to explain. Sometimes a waiter has noticed me struggling and brought a sharper knife to the table, not realising the problem. If a companion offers to cut the meat, I worry that their meal is getting cold while they help me, so I generally order meals that can be eaten with just the fork.

These are not just my little problems but those of so many people with arm problems - stroke victims, those with Parkinson's disease whose hands shake, and those with weak muscles. The embarrassment for people whose difficulties are not immediately obvious to those around them can cause acute problems and prevent them from eating out for fear of cutlery falling to the floor or flying across the table. Drinking may also be a problem. All the mishaps that might occur may cause other diners to laugh, not because they are unpleasant people, but simply through ignorance. It may also cause other diners discomfort. I long for greater awareness and understanding of disability – of the fact that some people need a little help to achieve the normality that the rest take for granted.

by Barbara Blackston Huntley

I think we have come a very long way since I was a child. I hope the improvements continue without either side losing a sense of humour about life and its ups and downs. Chips on shoulders do very little to improve life for ourselves or others, but making people aware that a problem exists sometimes brings about social change, albeit very slowly. Charities are generally very efficient at doing this today.

CHAPTER TWENTY

FREEDOM – AND PROBLEMS – AS THE CHILDREN GROW UP

A new "terror" awaited me when, exactly one year to the day after my first bone graft operation, I started working for HTI Engineering (formerly J & E Hall) on November 11, 1974. This was in an old office block in Hythe Street, Dartford, with very old-fashioned green metal desks and chairs. There was a paternoster lift which constantly went up on one side and down on the other. It was like a chain of open-fronted lifts that were always moving (except during breakdowns, which were frequent). The workers jumped on at one floor and off at another, often with arms full of papers. I was terrified at first of missing my footing and being jammed between lift and floor, but I soon got used to it. Even so, it was unpleasant if you forgot to jump off at the ground floor or the top floor. The chain of lifts went down into a totally dark brick housing at the bottom and, with a great clatter and shake, they moved across to the up side, where they eventually went into the roof space before clattering across the top and down again in a big loop. Even quite sane visitors sometimes believed the lifts turned on their side at the top and bottom of the loop; it was great fun to kid new people that this is what happened, so they were warned to make sure they jumped out in time!

The company's worldwide business was refrigeration and air conditioning. They did a lot of work in ships, breweries and cold stores. Business was booming and the offices were cramped with so many staff needed for all the procedures that were entirely manual then. We were shortly moved to a brand new office block built close by Dartford railway station to allow for expansion of the company and modernisation.

We all had lovely new wooden desks, modern facilities and a wonderful view across Dartford from the top floor, where I worked. The management hierarchy was still very male-orientated and women were very much second class workers, but things were slowly changing. The first sign of this was when management were expected to use the same dining area as the workers. Some of the men hated eating with clerks, secretaries and even people like handymen – but they got used to it or went elsewhere.

I liked my job in the Work-in-Progress section of Accounts. There was a great group of staff; we all enjoyed life and had a lot of fun.

We had a lively social life in local pubs at lunchtimes and in the evenings, when we would play darts. On one occasion, I organised a minibus trip to Brighton. We had a great day out, but on the way back the bus filled with smoke and everyone had to get out quickly. We were far out in the country, on a road with no phones, so I hitched a lift with the driver of an empty coach for some miles into Sevenoaks to get help. Another minibus was needed and we feared it would be a long time coming, so I rang my husband to ask him to let anxious partners know because they would be waiting at our destination. He then had to make the journey out to pick me up. He was not amused!

Our children now being older, Rod and I enjoyed a more active social life. We went fairly regularly to parties and dances and I found my new freedom very heady. I always felt I had missed out on being a 'wild' teenager, as my father had been so strict. Now I began to kick up my heels. Working had given me money to buy new clothes, improve my appearance from matronly Mum to something much more attractive. I wanted desperately to be thought modern and this was the era of the miniskirt (first time round) and ridiculously high platform soled shoes. I bought what I thought were young trendy clothes but which now look quite silly. I lost weight, but was never really slim. When I bent over in my very short skirts, others must have been amused or embarrassed – though I thought I was the 'cat's whiskers.' I frequently turned my ankles with my awful shoes.

Looking back, for the most part I thoroughly enjoyed life from the age of 27 to 45, apart from the two years of operations on my right hand. In October, 1975, I also had an operation on my left 'good' hand due to my fingers curling up. In 1980, I decided to learn to drive, but this was not going to be easy. Like my husband years before, I wanted to be sure I could drive before buying a car and having it adapted to drive with one hand. Drivers with arm disabilities seemed rarer than those with leg problems, so there was no way of getting tuition locally. However, I discovered that I could learn in London. Every Saturday morning, for many months, I travelled by train to Charing Cross, where an adapted Triumph Herald with automatic transmission was available.

On the day of my first lesson, I was both terrified and elated that at last I had the chance to become a driver. Would I ever make the grade? What would it be like learning to drive in London, where traffic was so heavy and taxi drivers were so dominant? As I sat on that train, I wanted to shout to everyone where I was going and what I was worried about. Often since then, I have looked at fellow travellers and wondered if their journeys might be a momentous day in their lives rather than the daily grind of travelling to work or business. For some it may be a trip to hospital, or maybe to meet someone new, or, like me, to do something they had never done before, all events which could change their lives. Our faces do not always mirror our minds.

When I reached the BSM office in Charing Cross Road, I was asked to wait until my instructor, returned with his last client; I was shaking as he arrived. He was an ex-ambulance driver who, I learnt, had the most amazing patience and understanding. He put me at ease at once and guided me out to the car, saying 'Don't worry, I will drive to a quiet street to begin your lesson.' I never realised there were so many quiet corners in London (perhaps there aren't any more), but my instructor knew plenty. I did not know where any of them were and could not have told anyone afterwards because I was so focussed on the car and what I was about to do.

When we reached a quiet spot, the instructor stopped the car and told me to get into the driver's seat. He talked me through the controls and then told me to start the car – 'put it into "drive," check the mirror and if it is safe to move off slowly, do so by putting your foot on the gas pedal.' I did not know the car ran on 'gas'! My blank look made him repeat 'Put your foot slowly on the accelerator.' This I did – only to be greeted with a blinding flash followed by a great clap of thunder. I visibly jumped, but managed to recover. Within a moment or two – omen or otherwise! - The heavens opened and we were in a tremendous rainstorm. John told me to brake gently to a halt (I am glad he had dual controls), and then he made sure I knew how to operate the wipers and lights with my one hand.

That lesson was mostly spent driving around a quiet London square to get me used to the controls. At the end, I felt absolutely drained - but I was eager to come back the next week. On my third lesson, I was given instructions to follow until I found myself driving around a very busy Hyde Park Corner. After this, I thought I was invincible. Rod joined me on my next lesson, but that was a disaster. He sat in the back, saying nothing (he was probably speechless with fear). They say pride comes before a fall and that lesson was about the worst I ever had. I drove appallingly and even attempted to overshoot a red light in Trafalgar Square, being saved by my instructor's foot on his brake. In his absence, some lessons were given by other instructors - but they seemed to have little knowledge of the disabled and I had little rapport with them. These lessons usually went badly.

My instructor eventually suggested I apply for my test, but when it came through it was in Gravesend, a town closer to my home. He suggested I cancel it and ask for another in London; otherwise, I would need to pay for hiring the car for six hours plus the test. But I was so keen to take it that I said I would pay. This was a big mistake - I had never driven in Gravesend and knew very little of the area. I failed miserably and returned with my tail between my legs for more lessons.

I reapplied and had a new test six weeks later in St. Johns Wood. I hadn't driven in that part of London, but had two lessons there before the test - and this time I passed. The examiner commented on how well I could drive; I could not believe it! It had taken nine months and some 45 lessons, but I had done it at last. On the train back, I wanted to tell everyone I had done it! I had my licence; I was free. Still full of excitement, I rushed home to tell my family: I had achieved my ambition. Shortly before passing my test, I had bought a second-hand Ford Escort estate car. It was now my pride and joy.

My children, meanwhile, were teenagers - with all the attendant problems for both parents and themselves.

Eventually, both children began work full-time and each was allowed to keep their first week's wage. After that, they were expected to contribute at least one third towards household expenses. Lee did not object, but he often borrowed money from us or his sister, which he was always made to pay back. He did not save and was generous when he had money. Krista was the opposite, saving and rarely borrowing. Nor did she like spending. Each attitude had its pros and cons. Loving both children dearly, I found it very hard trying to modify their contrasting faults - a merit with one was a fault with the other. Either can lead to problems.

My resolve was tested when Krista's salary was raised and I asked for more towards the housekeeping. She already considered the £6 she paid was far too much. She wanted independence and even threatened to leave home. Having led quite a sheltered existence until now, though, she was not very street-wise. So I was not particularly concerned, regarding it as an empty threat. How wrong I was! One day she came home and said: 'I'm leaving home; I've found a room in a house to share with two boys and another girl. My heart leapt. She could not be protected - she was vulnerable! What could I say?

'Oh, what is it like, dear?' I ventured.

'Well, I will have my own bedroom and we share all the other facilities, but they seem really nice people. Will you come and have a look at it with me?'

I realised it was better not to argue, as she would have to learn life's realities sooner rather than later, but I was very worried. Most of all, I wanted to stay her friend so that if things went wrong she could still turn to her parents without loss of face. This might have been awkward if we had disapproved. We went with her to see the house and its occupants. They were pleasant enough young people, but obviously more street-wise than our daughter. The house seemed clean and reasonably comfortable, but the bedroom for Krista was not a patch on her room at home -

which had just been expensively refurbished with fitted cupboards, new carpet, curtains and bedding.

The terms of her occupation were agreed and a date set for moving in. I suggested she just took her immediate requirements, with us bringing the rest once she was settled; in the meantime, if she did not like it, she could return home. However, I was very firmly told that she was taking everything she owned as she was tired of “keeping us all on her wages.”

I had my estate car, but had not passed my test when she moved out. It was ideal for packing all her belongings, so I drove it accompanied by Rod. It was dark and raining hard and the car was packed to the roof. I was very unhappy, but kept my feelings to myself.

We took her things up to the now empty bedroom - and I saw her face drop. The pictures formerly on the walls had been removed, leaving light marks and revealing how dirty the wallpaper was. The bare mattress of grey ticking looked sad and none too clean and the wardrobe and bedside cabinet were old and battered. Obviously, when our daughter had first seen the room, it had still been occupied and probably looked cosy with the bed made up and the previous occupant’s belongings in place.

I summoned a smile to say farewell to Krista, but I could tell she was starting to have doubts. I wanted to put my arms around her and say that if she felt it wasn't right for her she need not stay, but I knew I had to be strong for her sake. Escaping the nest is not always an easy option for either parents or children.

The next day, a Saturday, she phoned me and said she was not sure she would like it. I brightly said she should give it time. There was a hint of tears in her voice, but I pretended not to notice, I was longing to comfort her, but felt this was a lesson she had to learn the hard way. On Sunday she rang again, asking if she could come home. I suggested she give herself a fortnight to settle down, but to return then if she still felt the same way; she agreed reluctantly, but on Monday she rang from work, this time in tears and saying she would do anything, including paying more rent, if she could come home. I finally agreed, but said she must wait until the next day. On the Tuesday, Rod and I once again loaded the estate car to the roof for the return journey, and once again it was raining. It was a much chastened daughter who came back home; never again did she dispute the housekeeping she was asked to pay. I think in that one weekend she grew from a rebel into an adult.

Only once more did she cause any real concern as a teenager - when she suffered a broken romance. I felt her distress and so wanted to help because I knew she was deeply unhappy, but she rejected my efforts to console her; nothing I could do or say was acceptable. I could not get it through to her that the pain would ease; it made me feel a very incompetent mother. Of course she did recover. She met somebody else, Gary, who worked at the same company as her and her father; he too had suffered in the same way. They eventually married in August 1983. Krista stayed with us until her marriage and was a daughter to be proud of thereafter. The lessons we learned were hard for us both, but thankfully we emerged with our family relationship intact.

As for Lee, the problems Rod and I had with him stemmed from his earlier wanderlust - his constant desire to dabble in many things but to concentrate on few. He had been to college and got his City & Guilds qualification in welding and auto-engineering, which enabled him to get his first job as a trainee welder. However, he was never content for long and went from job to job, which was of great concern to me. For the most part, though, he did find his next job before leaving the last, and he was not afraid to go 'cold-calling' to find work.

When he was 18, I decided to throw a party for him at home. I baked and prepared everything, ordered a cake and invited the guests – some fourteen family and friends. I asked him to get home nice and early for the event – alas, he did not show up until 11.15 pm. He cut his cake, said 'hello' to everyone - and promptly went out again. I never forgave him for that - never again made a special effort for his birthday.

His romantic life seemed to follow his work pattern. I feared it would be many years before he settled, as he rarely seemed to have the same girlfriend for long. When he was 19 he met Sue, a young girl about 17 with whom he appeared very taken; I believe he saw her most days in the week following their first meeting. On the Friday of that week, Rod and I went out for a meal in the evening and on our return met our son getting out of a taxi with his new girlfriend.

'Come indoors quick, Mum and Dad,' he said excitedly. 'We've something to tell you!'

'Hold on a moment, I'm just going to put the car in the garage,' Rod replied.

'Well,' I said anxiously, 'she can't be pregnant; they've only known each other a week!'

When we got indoors, the young lady was proudly wearing a diamond solitaire engagement ring! 'My God,' I said, 'I'll have a whisky'.

I was shocked but I think I just said "Well I hope you will both be happy but you will have to work hard to save up to get married!"

I simply could not believe that it would last after such a hasty courtship. Once I got over the immediate shock, I wanted to do the right thing, but I was not prepared to buy a present for an engagement that I believed would not last. My solution was to open a building society account in my name and put in some money which would be theirs when they married. To their credit, they saved hard and tied the knot 17 months later in May 1980, when Lee was only 20. They have been married for over 34 years so I am happy to say I was wrong about their staying power.

I remember a work colleague saying to me: 'You must have been very upset when your son left home.'

'I have a flag flying from every window!' I jokingly replied. I must admit that it was a relief to know that I was no longer responsible for my loveable but very hyperactive son. I was always very worried and concerned for the children's problems, but once they were married I tried to avoid getting too involved. Rod and I would both offer any help we thought might be acceptable, but there were of course many times when we, as parents, had to stay quiet. My view is that families should try to preserve their bond through thick and thin. It is far from easy and only possible if all the members of the family feel the same way about the bond and allow the ties that bind them to overcome the problems that beset them. My roots and my family have always been of utmost importance to me.

CHAPTER TWENTY ONE

A NEW ERA – FOR BRITAIN AND ME

Nineteen-seventy-nine saw Margaret Thatcher's Conservatives sweep to power in Britain and this heralded a new era of push, push, push in the workplace. It was also not long before I landed a promotion that began a new chapter in my own life. In the work place, American ideas had crept in, with appraisals crucial to progression and everyone being expected to aim for the top. I was ambitious and fitted quite well into the new way of thinking. I was not attached to a union and felt quite capable of resolving my own battles to succeed in what was still very much a male-orientated environment. I had got promotion from Senior Clerk in Sales Ledger to an Overhead Controller looking after the manual accounts relating to all the expenses of running the company, at Hall Thermotank International Ltd, in Dartford (formerly J & E Hall. The company was always referred to locally as "Halls" even after many name changes. It has now gone from Dartford completely).

This department had a male manager and supervisor who, each morning it seemed, needed first of all to analyse any football games they had seen on TV the night before. There were days off for playing golf and these, too, would need to be discussed in detail before the day's work could begin. Then there was 'Page 3' of *The Sun* newspaper, with pictures of near-naked women to be reviewed. This all took time and we girls laughed at the way men moaned about women gossiping - they really should have heard themselves! Their chauvinism amused rather than annoyed us, but we felt sure they only put in 75% whilst we did 100%!

Then, of course, there were the office romances and the office vamp. Ours was a dark-haired young woman, small but well proportioned in all the right places. She would link arms with any passing male, open her eyes wide and flash her long black eyelashes seductively. The bright red lips would part as she cooed into her victim's ear, or loudly proclaimed her feelings for him. They either loved her or were acutely embarrassed by her, but no one could ever ignore her!

There was also the matron who had ruled the Petty Cash Office for many years and picked on the less fortunate members of staff for her verbal abuse. She unfortunately picked on me one day. Petty cash could only be claimed at certain hours of the day from a hatch in the Payroll Office. I went to claim my travel expenses and this forbidding lady turned her back to me, I waited an age while she ploughed through papers and cash on her desk without a word to me. At last, I asked if she would serve me as I had to return to my office.

'I've only got one pair of hands!' she shouted.

'And I have only three-quarters of a pair!' I replied saucily. She served me quickly and I was always served promptly after that.

The offices were always lively and when a young man was about to get married a number of gifts were piled high on the Divisional Manager's desk while he made a jokey speech to the gathered staff. The young man undid the parcels, one by one, until he came to the last - containing a spiked rubber condom. I, unfortunately, was standing next to a charming spinster lady nearing retirement who had obviously never seen or heard of such an item. 'What's that?' she asked innocently. 'It's just a fun thing.' I replied, hastily retreating across the office.

There were sad times, too. A lady in her 40s dreamed of becoming an actress. She was a great character, but somewhat naïve. She constantly sought our advice on problems in her life and in more personal things like make-up and clothes. She belonged to a drama group and her gestures were always dramatic, with lots of arm-waving and big smiles. Her long feline hands always had brightly-painted nails. We were all expected to read parts in any play she was learning and rehearsals were a very serious affair. She wore a tatty pair of sandals in the office, to which she was obviously very attached. The other girls would often hide these for fun, saying they had thrown them out, but she knew their tricks and would always find them. We all liked her even though we used to tease her a lot.

One day, as she was crossing the road after a rehearsal for her biggest performance, a French lorry came around the corner and ran over her, killing her instantly. I was first into the office next morning and the manager gave me the dreadful news. I could not believe that the lively, excited lady of the day before, who was so looking forward to her big chance, was no more. The office was silent for many days, the most poignant moment being when we cleared her desk and threw away those much-loved sandals. Somehow they epitomised her and their despatch brought tears to some eyes. Her funeral was very well attended; the bosses were among the mourners and the company flag flew at half mast. We all knew she would have loved the drama of it all.

When the sales ledger accountant left the firm, in late 1970s, I was promoted to his post. This was the start of a new era for me – twice over, in fact, coinciding with the first computers to be installed in the office. They had almost nothing in common with today's machines. All were linked to a huge central processing unit housed in a clean and locked department elsewhere. The machines on our desks were in no way interactive. They were merely tools to enter information into the system, replacing the bits of paper used by punch operators to input information into the central processor.

The day after the information was entered on a terminal screen, an error print run was produced on music-ruled continuous paper. This came back to the office with control totals and corrections were then made and the update followed the next day. By today's standards, the process was very laborious. Memory was very limited and access was by menu lists. Windows in those days were solely of the glass variety, not being used for access to computer programmes. We had never heard of 'Windows' with a capital W or PCs (except as constables in the Police force). There were frequent breakdowns and control was not easy; the system was not at all user-friendly. Computer programmers and analysts did not have a good relationship with the users and this caused serious problems at times because neither could understand the other. Clearly something had to be done to improve the worsening relations between the computer 'bods' and the workers.

In 1982 the company's solution was to buy an IBM System 38 computer for our department. A software house was appointed to write the programmes and the analysts moved in. This machine still had a central processing unit but was to be more interactive, giving people more access to the information they had input. I had written an up-to-date manual for the sales ledger, but there were no up-to-date ones for the other sections. This again left the software house with the problem of communication. Their efforts to write the software were also hampered by the lack of documentation; they soon became unpopular with the staff.

Management decided to get rid of all the staff at senior supervisor level from the accounts department and we were informed of this three months before the axe fell. This meant that I was among those about to be made redundant, but I think the fact that I had written a manual had made an impression on the newly-appointed manager of the systems department. I was offered a job as a systems analyst, to be the link between staff and programmers. This meant understanding both sides, testing the programmes and helping negotiate solutions to problems. It also meant travelling throughout the UK training regional staff to use the new programmes.

The job was very tough at first. There was a natural resistance to change, particularly in the likes of Glasgow, Avonmouth and Cornwall. From managers to foremen, all had run perfectly efficient manual systems; each saw no reason for change. I was resented as the person from Head Office Accounts poking her nose into their business and telling them how to run it. Gradually, though, they began to accept me and to appreciate the benefits of instant information. I tried to persuade them to see me as a helpmate in their learning process and a friend on the end of the phone for most of the time. I worked very long hours for no overtime pay and travelled hundreds of miles by train and plane, but I enjoyed what I did. I came to be accepted as the user's help in their hour of need. I suppose I was the forerunner of today's highly-organised help desks, but the relationship was much more personal. Many of those I met became appreciative friends, which I found very touching, but there was one region I never did manage to win over. That was Avonmouth. Right up to my last days with the firm, they were the authors of the most sarcastic and caustic memos I ever read! The manager there could not accept that a woman could be anything better than a good housewife and bedfellow, I felt that was the problem. I didn't fit his image of women!

Much though as I enjoyed my work with the users, management's growing arrogance towards them began to disillusion me. The attitude was becoming more hard line in the vein of 'if they don't like it, hard luck'. Programmers were regarded as the cream of the workers, but they understood very little of the problems that users might face when a programme did not work properly. I had to work closely with the programmers to test their output for the user. The long hours I gave to the company without overtime pay made me feel I should have a similar salary to theirs - their pay was some 25% more than mine.

In 1987, I approached my manager to ask for a higher salary. Her comment was that I could not have more pay, but at least I had the perk of staying in hotels and enjoying free meals. I did not see it as a "perk" to be living in hotels away from my family, being sent away at very short notice, providing my own business clothes, having to get up at 4 am to drive to the airport and not even being given a subsistence allowance. I had to account for my expenses to the very last penny, even for a newspaper. I often worked in my bedroom until 11 pm. I pointed all this out to my manager and said I would seek other work if I could not obtain better terms. She sensitively replied: 'At your age (49), and with your disability, you will find it very difficult to get another job'. That incensed me and I gave my notice in the next day!

When my manager had to report this to my director, she was told to ask what it would take to make me stay. It was explained that no more money was available for salary but I could name my price for living out. So the next day my manager apologised for her comments and it was agreed that I would stay.

I would be paid £28 living-out expenses plus have access to suitable training courses. So far so good, but from that day on I was never sent out again. It didn't really matter, for I had already made up my mind to seek another job.

I found one at The Woolwich Building Society in at their Head Office in Woolwich at a vastly increased salary and began there a few days before my 50th birthday. I was to implement a new Accounts Payable computer system. Working for a mutual building society (it became a bank after I left) was very different from working in industry, as I had done before. For one thing, they had begun to accept women in senior positions, although they still had an 'old boy' network that meant men met in the pub for informal business meetings. The atmosphere was starting to change and I could not believe that I was treated with so much respect and given so much support for any project I undertook. Nor was money any object, it seemed, because I was given all the equipment I asked for. Until now, I had always had to deal with tight budgets, mistrust and rejection of new projects. Respect had previously to be earned the hard way.

My staff comprised two young men and a supervisor who started one week after me. I had never had male staff before, but generally I found them very amenable and somewhat easier to control than young girls. There was no-one to show me the job because the previous Accounts Payable Controller had left three months earlier and the male clerks knew only the day-to-day procedures. So to some extent I was dependent on their goodwill. They were very helpful and never seemed to resent me personally, but I am sure there were times when it must have been irritating to be questioned by someone senior on how to do the job while I was trying to document the system.

Eventually, we all worked together as an excellent, growing team. After bringing in the new accounts payable system and designing a Society purchase order numbering system, I was promoted and moved into a separate office of my own. I trained the former supervisor to do my job and then wrote a computerised manual for the accounts payable system. I was proud to have proved that someone with a disability and few qualifications, and who was regarded by society as being 'old', could still achieve some success.

You never know what's round the corner, though, and in 1992 the Society decided that money was no longer freely available and that cutbacks were necessary. They asked for volunteers for redundancy or early retirement. The terms of the offer were excellent. With Rod planning to retire early in 1993 and with me suffering increasing health problems, I decided to volunteer. I left the Society after four-and-a-half years in the best job I ever had.

CHAPTER TWENTY TWO

UPHEAVAL AND DRAMA . . .
GOODBYE DANCING . . .
HELLO GRANDCHILDREN!

Back in 1980, meanwhile, Lee marrying and moving out had triggered a major re-think on the domestic front. Our house was very tatty, but we could see that with our son's departure we had at least gained a bedroom and lost a spare part store for cars – which is what his room had gradually become. I was also delighted to lose the smelly socks, the well-worn pullovers, the pin-ups, the car manuals, the dirty coffee cups, the coke cans and everything else that teenage boys collected at that time. Somehow the mess had seemed to overflow into the rest of the bungalow, so now I had dreams of a wonderfully clean and tidy house.

Rod and I made plans to improve the property. The trouble was, we rarely made the same plans but, after much arguing and negotiating, changes were agreed upon. Even so, we didn't realise what we were letting ourselves in for. The property was extended, causing a tremendous mess and upheaval. Dust filled our lungs from the knocking down of internal walls and seemed to get into everything else in spite of the dust sheets; we even felt as if we were eating it at times! There was nowhere to lay our heads for long, either, because the bungalow was been treated for woodworm and dry rot. The smell was awful and floorboards were up all over the place. We decided we needed to refurbish the whole place after the building work was completed.

Upheaval turned to drama, in more ways than one, in 1981. As well as passing my driving test, we completely redecorated our altered home and had almost finished when, in October, our first grandchild was born - a baby boy, Michael for Lee and Sue, much to our joy. We just had the hallway to finish papering and then the house job would be complete. Our traumas would shortly be behind us – or so we thought. In great excitement, we visited our new grandson and then, four days later, decided to go out with some friends to celebrate. But first Rod decided just to hang a couple of sheets of wallpaper. The ladder was leaning against the wall at one end of the hallway, but there was a high kitchen stool close to where Rod was working and he chose to stand on this. Big mistake. As he went to hoist himself up onto the stool, it overturned and sent him flying. He broke the femur of his polio leg, splitting the bone badly. He refused to let me call an ambulance, saying I could drive him to the hospital. He hopped, grey-faced, to my car.

At the hospital, I had trouble finding a wheelchair and then there was no-one to push it. I could not push with my paralysed right arm, so I pulled him through the double doors into casualty with my good left arm. It was very busy and we had a long wait. I was finally told to take him to X-ray. Still there was no-one to push, so I zigzagged the wheelchair along the wide corridor from left wall to right wall until I reached the X-ray department. It must have looked very funny - but it was all very painful for Rod. His leg had to be pinned right through his knee. Because we had eaten a curry meal that evening, he could only have a local anaesthetic. Rod already had dents on either side of his knee where it had been pinned as a child when he had polio. The surgeon used the same dents to place a pin through his knee. Rod then spent a month in hospital in traction and a further six months at home recovering.

Ten days after Rod's accident, disaster struck again. I was driving Krista to Gravesend on a Christmas shopping trip when I was hit by a van that went into the back of my estate car; fortunately we escaped injury. The insurance was in Rod's name. I was dreading going to the hospital to tell him what had happened, but he took it very well. I was glad when the year came to an end and hoped 1982 would be a bit less dramatic.

After two weeks' convalescence in The Wellcome Foundation's beautiful home overlooking Poole harbour, Rod returned to work in May, 1982. Alas, our dancing days were now behind us. We had been going to his firm's dances every two or three weeks and really enjoyed meeting all our friends there, but his leg was never quite so strong again. We tried a few times to dance, but could never recapture the magic of those few previous years.

Nineteen-eighty-three was another notable year, both happy and sad. We had the added joy of a second grandson, Gavin, the death of my beloved father and the excitement of our daughter's wedding.

My father died just a few days after I had learned that he had leukaemia. What neither my mother nor I had realised was that my father's sight was failing; he had wanted no-one to know. He stopped reading the newspapers or books that he had so enjoyed. When my mother queried this, he just said he could not be bothered to read. He began to smoke again, which he had not done for three years. My mother greatly missed the car (she could not drive) and I think the quality of their lives began to deteriorate. A sort of sadness crept in – a realisation that the most pleasant part of their lives, their retirement years when they were still active, was coming to an end.

My father's death was three weeks after a happy weekend in Bournemouth, but I blamed myself for taking him away when the weather was so cold and windy. Had I killed him? I asked myself. Consolation only came when I later read a very brief note in his diary: 'WONDERFUL WEEKEND.' He usually only wrote down his engagements, without comment. I was so glad he had enjoyed his trip and greatly comforted by this comment.

My mother and I visited the undertakers to make the funeral arrangements – which had a lighter moment. The lady there said my father's death had to be registered in the area of the hospital where he died. I said I did not know the area and asked for directions, only for Mum to interject: 'Oh, don't worry, your Dad knows the way!' Poor Mum, I did not know whether to laugh or cry. 'I don't think he will be able to tell us the way, Mum,' I said gently.

She laughed: 'I am silly; for a moment, I had forgotten he is no longer here.' Sadly, it was a very long time before she laughed again. I have greatly missed my father ever since. He had a quiet manner and a caring attitude. He suffered much pain. He was hardworking, intelligent and had a great sense of humour. He was in the eyes of the world an ordinary man, but to me he was a colossus whose example I can never live up to.

Life moved on. With my two grandsons, I found great joy and love. I adored being a grandmother; it is so much less stressful than being a parent. You know the ropes you've 'been there, done that and got the T-shirt.' You can have a spoil without feeling you are ruining the child's upbringing. Rod and I loved the holidays, weekends and evenings when we could have them after work. There is something very satisfying about teaching a small child the basics of life, like counting, colours, shapes and letters, but not just those things. I loved to talk to them about the world around them, the trees, the plants, the fields, rivers and the stars. We loved to play games in the garden, grandparents shouting as loud as the little ones. We danced and sang around the living room and as they grew older I had great fun teaching them to cook. We made lots of cakes, advancing to bread, pancakes, pizzas and a fully-fledged dinner for their parents one evening when we made chefs' hats for them to wear. They shopped for and prepared the whole meal themselves, finally serving the family. Michael, my elder grandson started at catering college in 1998 and I like to think I had a small part in his enthusiasm for a career in catering. Unfortunately the unsocial hours and low wages meant he did not stay in the catering industry for long, but I think he does a lot of cooking for his wife and two children.

We went on picnics, to the parks and many other places of interest, but the grandchildren also learned that life was not fun for everyone. Their great-grandparents needed love and care because sometimes they could not care for themselves - especially Rod's mother, who was now a house-bound invalid, with us doing her washing and shopping every week. Michael and Gavin often accompanied us to see her every week.

It wasn't all sweetness and light between the boys and Rod, who tended to be rather stricter than I was. At meal times, he expected nothing left on the plates. Faddyness was not encouraged and dislikes not easily tolerated. Perhaps his views were the result of a wartime upbringing in a very poor family when, if you disliked the food, there was nothing else to eat and you went hungry.

I dreaded the battle of wills that mealtimes could become. I remember Gavin, just two, refusing to eat his meal and Rod roaring: 'You will sit on that chair until the food is eaten and will not leave the table until I say so.' The child puffed his cheeks out, pursed his lips and stared very hard and long at his grandfather. The look said: 'You will not intimidate me, nor will I eat this food.' Gavin did not speak, but the look grew more baleful until, some 15 minutes later, he tried to get down from the table.

'Get back on that chair until I say you can get down,' said Rod firmly. His grandson silently got back on the chair, but the stare had become evil! Further attempts were made to get down, but the battle lasted almost an hour until I quietly interceded with Rod, feeling that it had gone on too long and was now at stalemate. 'Right! You may leave the table now,' I said, 'but you had better behave or you will be made to sit on that chair again until bedtime!' The small boy left the table with some dignity and, with his hands behind his back, marched over to his grandfather. He stood firmly in front of him and, with as much venom as he could muster, shouted: 'RAT BAG!!' I am afraid I giggled as I rather shared his sentiment, but even Granddad was forced to smile.

CHAPTER TWENTY THREE

DEATH AND LIFE

Life can be so cruel, and a family tragedy in January, 1988, hit me hard. We were all looking forward to the birth of Krista's first child. She had a very happy pregnancy. At 2.30 a.m. one morning, with the birth imminent, our phone rang. I jumped out of bed, wondering: is it a girl or boy! 'Mum, it's me.'

'News?' I said.

But a great sob came down the line as my daughter said: 'Mum, I've lost the baby!'

'Oh no,' I gasped 'do you want us to come to the hospital now?'

Rod and I, numbed, drove through the dark and windy streets, which fortunately were largely deserted. The tears streamed down my face as I thought: 'This is a nightmare, I will wake in a moment, this can't really be happening; it's a good pregnancy with no problems.'

We were taken into the labour ward, where Krista lay with Gary sitting ashen beside her and holding her hand tightly. We were not prepared for the sight of our dear little granddaughter in a cradle beside the bed and I thought: 'Oh thank God, it was a mistake and she is not dead.' The peaceful little face looked so beautiful with gorgeous auburn curls. She had asphyxiated during birth, but was perfect. I was distraught for Krista and Gary's suffering. It seemed so unfair that such a wanted child, with so much love awaiting her, had not had the chance of life.

The way Krista and I dealt with our grief was quite different. I wanted to scream and shout; I was angry, hurt and helpless to remove the pain. Krista was silent and for the most part grieved inwardly. She did not want to share her feelings and was outwardly very calm. I wanted to share her pain and give love and support. Being able to comfort your own child is what most mothers want to do when things go wrong, but I felt totally inadequate as I stayed with her. We held hands and the tears were never far away, but neither of us could express our feelings to the other as I so wished we could have done.

Kind people sent flowers to Krista and Gary, but the house became so full of them that Krista felt overwhelmed. I suppose they prevented normality, stopping the pretence that this was not happening. Krista agreed that anyone who suggested sending flowers be asked to make a donation instead - to the hospital towards the purchase of a monitor for mothers in labour. If one had been fitted to Krista, my granddaughter might have lived. We hoped that when the monitor was bought it would save other lives.

For my part, the hurt I felt for Krista and the loss of her baby affected me very badly. She and Rod are resilient people, neither inclined to discuss sad or morbid events, but I wanted someone to talk to. I felt constrained. I was in a new job – as an Accounts Payable Controller with The Woolwich Building Society at their recently opened new offices in Bexleyheath, Kent. So I had few friends there who were close enough for me to express my personal feelings, whilst other friends were either too far away or not very close to me mentally. My grief, I am ashamed to say, took the form of anger when I looked in prams at other women's babies. Why did they have what my daughter could not have? My thoughts were totally unreasonable, but I doubt if I am alone among grandparents who have suffered in this way.

The pain slowly eased and life had to move on. The sad memories remained, but intruded less in daily life. For us, the sun shone again 18 months later when Krista gave birth to a beautiful healthy, dark-haired daughter, named Natasha, and then, two-and-a-half years later, a beautiful blue-eyed blonde girl named Danielle, joined the family.

My grandchildren have been a tremendous joy to me, I just hope that one day they will experience the love and pleasure that my whole family has given me, I fear they will also have to experience the traumas too, I hope they will have the courage to face them.

Life also goes on through other means. In October, 1987 – three months before Krista's tragedy - we awoke one night to the hurricane that caused devastation across southern England.

by Barbara Blackston Huntley

Countless beautiful trees came down. My personal feelings led me to ask The Wellcome Foundation if I might purchase an English oak sapling to plant in the grounds of Acacia Hall in Dartford. Permission was granted and in November that year - on my 50th birthday - my young grandsons, Michael and Gavin aged 5 and 3 joined me with small spades to plant the little tree up on a raised grassy bank. I love the great English oaks and hope that one day my ashes will rest beneath one. I wondered whether 'my' tree would grow to great heights; it was only my height (about 1.5 metres) when I planted it, but is now about 12 metres high. My dream is that one day it will be a huge old oak, although I rather fear that the ground upon which it stands may one day be built upon. It no longer belongs to The Wellcome Foundation but to the local Dartford Borough Council who have refused to put a preservation order on the oak tree. It stands on a bank beside the river Darent (Celtic meaning of the word is "a river where Oak trees grow") now in Hesketh Park, Dartford, by a bridge dedicated to the local EllenorLions Hospice.

CHAPTER TWENTY FOUR

CARING AND RETIREMENT

As we moved into the 1990s, the seriously declining health of Rod's mother and her older sister were a growing cause of concern, frustration – and, I admit, a sense of guilt. My mother-in-law now needed constant care. Pathetically bent over a little wooden trolley, she could not walk more than a few steps at a time. Social Services arranged to send Joan, a wonderful carer, to prepare her meals, look after her personal needs and do some housework during the week. She had to be put to bed in the evenings and had a stream of other carers for evenings and weekends. She dearly loved her "Joanie," but hated not knowing who would come when Joan was unavailable.

Rod and I visited her often, shopping and washing and taking her out when we could or having her to stay, but it was becoming very difficult for us. I could not push her wheelchair with my one good hand and Rod and I both struggled to get her into the car. It was so painful, with her arthritic limbs, to heave her down the steps from her front door into our car. My damaged back and Rod's inability to balance properly on his two legs, because of his polio, only added to our difficulties. To get her into the car or bed when she stayed, we lifted and pushed as best we could and she gritted her teeth - but the situation steadily worsened. I felt guilty that we were not coping very well. We were also caring for her older sister, who had similar problems but was not in such a bad way at first. Both women were in their late 80s, of a very independent nature, and both sometimes fell out of bed.

They were connected to a Piper Lifeline System attached to a local authority control centre, who would always contact us when they fell as they both lived alone. When the phone rang, we would leap from our bed and dress quickly, jump in the car and get to their homes as fast as we could. We usually found them huddled on the floor and had to get them back to bed as best we could. Sometimes it happened twice in a night. It was as difficult for them as it was for us, but neither lady was prepared to go into a home. By the end of 1991, both Mother-in-law and her sister, Elsie, were in different hospitals at the same time. It was New Year's Eve and Elsie's hospital decided they wanted to discharge her - but no care could be arranged as it was holiday time.

This was turning into a nightmare. We were trying to visit both, but we also had jobs to go to. Both were eventually discharged and we muddled along as before for about a month. Then we found Mum B unable to get out of bed - but she refused to go into hospital. I was desperate. There was nowhere for us to sleep in her house and no central heating, and she would not eat. I called her doctor and two days later, when pneumonia set in, she finally agreed to return to the local cottage hospital. Her condition rapidly worsened and we believed death was near, but she was transferred to the general hospital, eventually recovering and being sent home. Her indomitable spirit had won through once again.

I was intensely frustrated with my situation and felt guilt because I knew going into a home was unacceptable to both women. I understood their feelings, but resented their apparent failure to understand that Rod and I felt we could no longer cope with the worry of not knowing how they were to be cared for if we could no longer lift them. I was getting frequent calls at work and at home from about them both when a carer did not turn up, or when their regular carers were unavailable. I dealt with their bills such as rent, council tax, and forms they could not complete, of which there were many, but the pressure of their problems was getting to me. I also had my own elderly mother who, unknown to her, had Parkinson's disease. She felt resentment that I was obliged to care for my in-laws and thought other people should recognise my problems.

I dearly loved them all. I had tremendous admiration for their stoicism in the face of adversity, their toughness and their determination, but I felt as if I was drowning because no-one in the family understood the growing demands upon me - doing a full-time job, caring for grandchildren and running my own home.

Mentally, I was not coping at all well. Sometimes I wished I could just walk away from it all. I wished I could talk to someone who could understand the isolation I felt. I am sure many others have felt just as I did at that time. I knew most of my in-laws' physical needs were being met by Social Services, but my mental strain grew daily.

Some years later, when I was in hospital myself, I found many people there who were coping with little or no proper care in the community because all our welfare needs are governed by the availability of cash. I met a lady living in an iron lung; she was totally paralysed and unable to do anything at all for herself, unable even to breathe alone. Her local authority said they had insufficient money to provide the 24-hour care her doctors said she needed. Her choice was to receive only five hours of care in 24 hours or go into a home and live away from the husband she loved, who was also disabled.

Families are rarely self-supporting now, as they were when I was a child. They have fewer aunts, uncles, brothers, sisters, children to provide a network of care and support. All adults are expected to work, including mothers of school-age children and the disabled - unless such disability is severe. Retired people who are living longer, but whose quality of life has deteriorated, do not want to enter homes - but relatives who care for them are often grandparents themselves. They may also be caring for grandchildren, whilst their children are doing full-time jobs. Those who stay at home from choice are often regarded by society as second rate or rich.

What will happen to future generations now both men and women are expected to work until they are 67 or older? Will working grandparents still be expected to support their older and younger families or will society develop a professionally efficient social support network at an affordable price? The early 21st Century has freed us with technology to shop from our homes (and even control them from mobiles) but has not yet found a solution for our aging population. Those who do not have the capacity to use computers are now un-catered for by our society. Now in my late 70s I fear for my future and the disabled fear for their lives and well-being. I would prefer death to being in a home where profit is the criteria for running it. Governments may recognise the problems and want to change things, but social change only seems to come about quickly if disaster strikes, as it did in the 1939-45 war. Mostly, it is a very slow process.

By 1992, my own physical well-being was a growing concern. The late effects of polio were affecting my ability to drive and to use a keyboard for long periods. My overworked left arm was very painful at times from inflammation of the tendons. I had arthritis in my wrist, neck and spine and very sudden swelling of the wrist and hand due to rheumatism. Rod planned to retire early in April, 1993, and I had planned to leave work about the same time. We wanted to see something of the world before we got too old or infirm, but my pain persuaded me to leave more than a year earlier.

I approached my manager, who was very understanding. He said he did not want to lose me and suggested I could take a medical break if my doctor felt a rest would help - after which I could return. This was duly arranged, but before I took the break The Woolwich (then still a building society) decided they needed to cut back. For the first time ever, they asked for volunteers for redundancy/early retirement. I decided this was a good opportunity, so I volunteered and was allowed to go in July, 1992.

The time I spent at home before Rod retired felt like a holiday. It was good to catch up on all the things I had wanted to do but never had the time. I still had my car and when my arm was not too painful I could take myself out and have lunch with friends or go shopping. I really enjoyed that year and began to recover from my negative feelings. I felt almost young again (I was 54), my health improved without the pressure of work and I was on top of the world. Rod was welcomed home to more creative menus and life seemed very pleasant. The difficulties of caring for Rod's mother and her sister now became easier as I had more time to cope with their growing problems. I joined a Spanish class, which I enjoyed very much, although I don't think I will ever manage to do much more than order a meal or read the labels in shops.

As for those travel plans, Rod and I decided we simply could not wait . . .

CHAPTER TWENTY FIVE

MAGICAL EXPERIENCES ON THE OTHER SIDE OF THE WORLD

For our first long trip – starting on 16 August, and lasting until the 4 September 1993 - we chose the Canadian Rockies and Alaska. It was a wonderful experience to see the wildness of the Rockies, the huge mountain ranges towering high into skies that were sometimes deep blue and at other times menacingly black, with the mountain tops disappearing into the clouds. We flew over great ice fields, walked on glaciers gleaming in the sun and gazed into crevasses of blinding blue ice. We saw valleys with meandering grey/blue streams covered in rock flour ground down by the glaciers as they moved over the mountains. In Alaska we saw and heard the thunderous roar of a glacier carving into the sea. We marvelled at chipmunks, bears, elk and salmon spawning.

This trip whetted our appetite for travel. Luckily, we could afford more of the same – thanks to our simple lifestyle at home, our lifetime habit of saving and our joint redundancy money. Our second long haul was a six-week trip in 1995, starting with the bustle of Hong Kong before its return to China. It was noisy and cramped and smelled of sweetness and drains; at night, it was a kaleidoscopic mass of lights and colour. We left in a typhoon from the old Kai Tak airport, where the short runway was sandwiched between skyscrapers. It was lashed by wind and rain and we were soaked to the skin, but the pilot did a fantastic job in getting off the ground. Very scary, though!

Our next stop was Singapore, which was very hot and humid. This was just a brief overnight job, but we were struck by the excellent and efficient service from everyone - from airport to hotel and on the trip and then back to the airport for our flight to Australia. We landed in Cairns at 7.30 am. with jet lag making us feel like zombies, but we soon recovered to enjoy the wide open spaces of Down Under. We visited The Great Barrier Reef, which to us was an 'out of this world' experience. Rod went snorkelling and I saw the corals from a little submersible glass-bottomed boat. It was a truly rare and wonderful experience to see the great variety of multi-coloured corals and the huge giant clams with electric blue eyes like great dashes of light.

We took a four-wheel drive over dirt roads and rocky river beds on a crocodile safari, but the crocodiles were few. We saw only one small one, although stories abounded of humans coming to grief on the river banks! We drove to the rain forest of the east coast, where we saw great rattan vines (woody climbing plants). Our guide told us that we were to beware of the 'wait-a-while' vine; we soon found out why. These vines have barbed hooks, a little like fishhooks. They can catch in your clothes and skin - and you have to 'wait a while' to be freed!

A very old train, once used to transport the gold-diggers, hauled us up to Kuranda, a mountain retreat village. Then we joined a cable car to fly high above the rainforest. It was literally a 'bird's eye view.' I was spellbound as we drifted silently over the huge dense green canopy of trees and great waterfalls below. The balmy air caressed our faces through the open window. People looked so far away and insignificant in this place, where nature seemed to reign supreme. I hoped no-one would talk; I just wanted to melt into the forest and the sky above.

Back on terra firma, we visited the old telegraph station in Alice Springs and the School of the Air, where we heard lessons being conducted with children of the Northern Territories. This was also the operations centre of the Flying Doctor service. A five-hour drive from Alice Springs took us to Ayers Rock in the red centre of Australia. We experienced sunset and sunrise - we got up at 3.45 am for the sunrise - but I was disappointed. For me, it was neither a spiritual nor a magical experience. I felt the stories about the rock were probably more hype than truth. The tremendous heat and the flies that seemed desperate to invade noses, mouths and eyes added to my dislike of what, to me, was just a huge lump of rock sticking up out of a flat sea of red sand and shrub.

New Zealand had the sort of scenery I really enjoyed - rolling hills, craggy mountains and caves - but the experience I will never forget was a helicopter flight to the top of the Franz Josef Glacier just before bad weather set in. The clouds rolled down the mountain, blotting out everything and forcing the cancellation of further trips. Rod had not wanted to come, but I was very excited by the prospect of repeating my Canadian experience. The helicopter pilot put us down in the soft snow on top of the mountain and we got out, sinking into the virgin whiteness all around. The scenery was utterly breathtaking. The cold fresh air was exhilarating, but the black clouds were rolling along and beginning to make the pilot nervous. He urged us back into the helicopter and took off quickly, almost tipping the machine on its side as he flew down the rugged side of the mountain. We were looking straight down into what seemed like bottomless blue crevasses – all very exciting!

From New Zealand, we flew to Fiji and sailed around the little Yasawa Islands in a motor yacht. The all-male Fijian crew cooked our simple meals, which we ate in the back of the open boat or on the beaches. One day we watched as they wove coconut palm leaf envelopes in which to place the food for a lovo feast the next day of chicken, pork, lamb, fish and sweet potatoes. A fire was started in a hole dug in the ground. When the flames subsided and the wood and coals were red hot, rocks were placed on top and the woven baskets of meat placed on these. The food was covered with sacks and then a good layer of sand and cooked for about five hours. When this was complete, the ship's cook and his boy dug out the food from the burning hot sand, on which they walked in their bare feet.

Another memorable event was a Yaqona welcoming ceremony by the villages of Nacula Island. We went ashore in a little boat, paddling the last few yards onto the golden sand. We walked through the coconut palms at the back of the beach, and there was Malakati village. Some of the houses were rather dilapidated grass huts – Buras - and a few were concrete block houses. At one end of the village, the raised chief's house was made of palm with a magnificent thatched roof and patterned walls. At the opposite end was a church that was sadly in need of repair. The people were very poor, with little to spend on their homes or surroundings. Even so, they were the happiest people we met in all our travels, with huge welcoming grins. Their pleasure at seeing us was all too obvious as they garlanded us with leis of frangipani flowers, giving off the most wonderful scent.

Inside the church, our cruise director explained the local customs and the Karva ceremony, in which we were about to join. Men and women were not permitted to wear hats or to take photos without permission because some of the locals believed it destroyed their souls. Men were to precede women and sit cross-legged on the grass in front of the chief, his assistant and the mayor. Women had to sit at the rear. No-one should raise their head above that of the chief. We learnt that Fijians regard the human head as sacred - it must not be touched by other people.

The chief and his assistants prepared a dish of Karva (a type of capsicum pepper root) in a huge wooden bowl. It looked like brown mud and was offered to each of us in half a coconut shell. We were expected to drink it straight down, but it was **the** most disgusting taste! Within a few minutes, our lips and tongue were numb - a very strange feeling.

The rest of the ceremony was quite delightful, with the villagers singing and dancing for us in their grass skirts. The singing was the most melodious I ever heard and the dancing was vigorous and exciting. The men brandished spears and dashed towards us as if they would run through us – only to stop at the last moment and flash their huge grins before whirling off again.

Afterwards, they danced with us. This was quite amusing as Rod's polio leg does not perform too well on a dance floor. It behaved even worse on the coarse grass here! A young girl had asked him to dance with her and she was full of giggles as her whole family gathered at the door of their hut to watch and laugh at the performance. All of the people were openly very curious about our polio limbs, but their curiosity was in no way offensive.

The Fiji experience reminds me of a more recent holiday in the Seychelles, when we visited a very primitive village on the island of Nosy Bé, which is part of Madagascar. The people here were desperately poor, living in grass huts on stilts. They produced the most beautiful embroidered table cloths and I was curious how they kept them so white in the heat and dust of the village where there were no roads, just tracks through the huts and the surrounding forest leading to the beach. As we walked through the village in our shorts and sleeveless tops, everyone seemed fascinated by the distorted limbs of Rod and myself. There were no beaming smiles here, but the curiosity was the same; everyone stared hard, but again it was somehow inoffensive. We were surrounded by children who followed us to the beach. There the boys wanted to sell us small boats they had carved and the girls offered little tray cloths they had embroidered. We swam and then sat among the children, playing with the little ones and communicating by writing our names in the sand or trying a few words of French; they spoke a kind of Patois French.

The children followed once more as we left the beach and a girl of about 13 linked arms with Rod. 'I think I've got a girlfriend!' he said to me. She obviously understood and went into gales of giggles. I looked behind at the dozen or so children following and discovered they were all walking along imitating Rod's pronounced limp! I hoped the travellers on the next ship that called at the island did not find a village populated by limping children!

Gradually the health of my in-laws, now in their 90s, had deteriorated to the point where I could not lift them and cope with frequent falls that eventually broke their bones and there was no other alternative for their care except in nursing homes. I could not sleep, thinking about their feelings and worrying about their situation. Both eventually died. There were few to mourn them. These two women were both tough, hard-working, courageous, unsung women, like so many of their generation. They had faced two world wars, poverty and poor housing conditions. They had few rewards, but never complained; in fact, both had seemed very content with their lot until they had to enter homes.

The way their lives ended has frightened me a great deal. I don't want to go out that way. I fear I will lack their strength and fortitude. I don't know whether we should have the right to choose our end if life becomes unbearable, but I find it a very troubling thought. To combat my negative feelings – while my mother-in-law and her sister were still alive in homes - I had decided to do some voluntary work. For a short while, I helped in the library of a local technology college. When that ended, I approached the local Volunteer Bureau, who suggested I might be suitable for the local Citizens Advice Bureau (CAB). I was interviewed and attended an assessment day, after which I was accepted for training. This was quite a lengthy process, attending courses and studying both in the Bureau and at home. So it was nine months before I was able to interview clients. Volunteers had to commit themselves to at least six hours' work each week and attend ongoing training courses.

I worked at the CAB for almost three and a half years and thoroughly enjoyed what I did, although it was both exhausting and emotional at times. We dealt with a whole range of human problems such as benefits, debt, divorce and separation, housing, employment, consumer, utilities, disability, legal, racism, domestic violence, homelessness and many others too numerous to mention. Often people are advised by benefits agencies, courts and magazines and newspapers to contact us for advice. It is given free to everyone who needs it and the general advisors are all unpaid, although the manager and some specialist advisors may receive remuneration. Funding is always a problem, particularly in poor areas - which is often where the need is greatest.

CHAPTER TWENTY SIX

AN EVENTFUL START TO THE NEW CENTURY

Talk about starting the new Millennium with a bang. That was almost literally the way of it. We duly cheered as the 21st Century began at midnight on the December 31, 1999, with everyone hoping the New Year would be happy and healthy. Just hours later, though, I woke up feeling terribly unwell. At first I just put it down to over-celebration – but it seemed every bone in my body was aching and my head was throbbing. Within hours I was back in bed, and there I stayed for four days with severe influenza.

Then I thought I felt better. I went to the bathroom, but as I rose from the toilet seat I collapsed onto the bathroom floor. When I regained consciousness, I realised I had once again broken my polio arm – for the 3rd time in my life. This arm has no muscle in its upper part, so it was skewed at a very odd angle. My scream caused poor Rod to wake from a deep slumber. He called an ambulance and I spent the next week in hospital. It was not normal practise to plaster a break in the humerus bone, but I knew my arm would not heal without it; the broken bone was totally unstable without surrounding muscle. I was in hospital for almost a week before I was allowed to speak to the consultant. Fortunately, he had worked at The Lane Fox Unit of St Thomas' Hospital and had some experience of polio and its late effects. He arranged for the arm to be plastered and then I was sent home.

The plaster was very heavy and, as I have no shoulder muscles to hold the bone into the shoulder blade, the ligaments to my arm were almost torn out of my shoulder. The pain was excruciating. In the middle of the night, my husband took me to an emergency doctor who gave me morphine and the next day I was sent to the fracture clinic. Here I saw the consultant again and he arranged for a lightweight brace to be put on my arm. I was in that brace for four months.

by Barbara Blackston Huntley

My mother had reached her 90th birthday in 2000 and was living in sheltered accommodation in Beckenham, which was at times a difficult drive for Rod and me. We did her shopping each week and Rod was finding this difficult as his paralysed leg was getting weaker. Mum, too, needed more care than we could give at a distance. So when a bungalow became available close to our home, I thought it might be the solution for both of us if she moved. She agreed and negotiations began in earnest to buy the property. The chain for sale of her flat and purchase of her bungalow was a very worrying time for me as the seller of the bungalow was 91 and going into a nursing home; the buyer of Mum's flat was 89 and of course Mum was well into her 90th year. I worried what would happen if one of them in the chain departed this life before completion, which took six months due to many problems with both sale and purchase. We did reach the end with everyone still breathing, although at times I felt I might be the one who did not make it as the experience was very traumatic!

Mum settled down reasonably well in her new home, but missed her old friends in the sheltered accommodation. I cared for her as best I could, cooking her meals and doing her washing as she grew less able. Sometimes I bought her a little treat and one day I bought her a raspberry cheesecake. The next day I asked her if she enjoyed it. 'Oh no,' she said. 'I put it on my salad for lunch and didn't enjoy it at all!'

'It was a dessert, why did you put it on your salad?" I asked.

'Well, you said it was cheese!" Obviously, cheese to Mum was always a savoury dish.

Before Mum moved, I decided I wanted to work with children after spending so much time caring for my elderly relations. I applied to a local primary school to help as a volunteer with reading. I had an interview and they seemed keen to have me, but the procedure was long drawn out. It meant I had first to give them a CV, have a criminal records check, a report from my GP, a personal reference and a reference from my previous employers. I managed to get through all the hoops and began work. The children were of all levels of intelligence - some were competent readers, some barely able to recognise their letters. I thoroughly enjoyed being with them, but in the wake of the Soham murders no volunteers were allowed to be alone in a room with a child. (In August 2002 two ten-year-old girls were killed in the village of Soham, Cambridgeshire, with a caretaker at the local secondary school subsequently convicted.)

Instead of me being in a room with a child, we had to sit in a corridor. This was a very noisy place as classes frequently changed lessons and curious children noisily interrupted our reading together. 'Wha ya doin?" was frequently asked. The voices of each class of five- to 11-year-olds passing behind our chairs were not the only distraction; often a pupil I was helping would be thumped, or a hand would reach out to the book or game being used. The more vicious children pulled the hair or ears of the unfortunate pupil sitting beside me.

After I had been doing this work for a while, I was asked if I would like to train with VRH (Voluntary Reading Help). This was an organisation devoted to training people to work with children who have learning difficulties, especially with reading. I trained for six months and was assigned to help three boys individually – at the same school where I had already been working, The Brent Primary School in Dartford - not only with reading but also with playing board games and discussing their interests. We were given a box of books and games, but I often found more in charity shops. One boy was slightly autistic, one had brain damage from a road accident and one was a hard-nosed tearaway who hated reading. My greatest success was with the tearaway; after two years, his form teacher told me he was actually asking to read books. The key was his love of sport, particularly books about football, so I took those magazines in and he wanted to read them.

Another boy was extremely disruptive in the classroom and the bane of all the teachers' lives. He was constantly being sent out of the classroom to sit in the corridor. One day he sat in an alcove behind where I was working with another child. I felt something lightly hit the back of my neck, but thought it must be a fly so brushed my neck. A little later it happened again, only much harder and I realised this seven-year-old was throwing something at me. I called him over and asked: 'What have you got in your pocket?'

'Nothing.'

His pocket was bulging. I asked him to turn it inside out. A shower of tiny dried macaroni shells fell to the floor. He had been pinging these with great accuracy at the back of my neck. I later discovered he could read much better than most of his classmates. He was bored when he was not stimulated by the work being done in his class. He was very intelligent, but the class had so many children with learning difficulties it seemed the work was geared more to their needs than those of the brightest pupils.

My main responsibility now, though, was my mother and I went in to her new home every day to sort out problems and to see that she could heat up her pre-cooked meals. She had a man friend who took her out to lunch once a week, but one day when she was unwell I said I would prepare something for them both. I had cooked an apple pie, which I said she would just need to warm in her Baby Belling oven. Next day I asked if they enjoyed the pie. 'That oven is no good!' she said. 'It burnt the top of your pie black and the bottom was still cold!' I checked and found it was set to Grill; she had used the wrong switch.

I grew accustomed to her strange attempts to feed herself, but her breakfast one morning in her 93rd year was truly life-changing. She normally had corn flakes for breakfast, but she read in a magazine that raisins soaked in gin were very good for arthritis. Overnight, she soaked the raisins in some gin, but by morning they had absorbed the liquid and so she added her corn flakes and poured on more gin. She seemed quite cheery when I saw her later in the day and Rod and I laughed about it. Next morning I found her on the floor; her legs were paralysed. She never walked again and after hospital treatment she ended up in a nursing home for the rest of her life.

CHAPTER TWENTY SEVEN

GROWING CHALLENGES . . .
MORE JOY AND GRIEF . . .
LEARNING, DOING, HELPING

"**While polio is essentially a disease of the past, an increasing number of people who have had polio are developing a condition called post-polio syndrome (PPS).** PPS is a poorly understood condition that can cause a variety of symptoms, including pain, muscle weakness and fatigue."

I quote from the National Health Service website. PPS has increasingly become a factor in my own life and in 2001 it led to my referral to the Lane Fox Respiratory Unit of St Thomas' Hospital, the only unit of its kind in the UK. PPS was beginning to be recognised in people who had suffered poliomyelitis many decades earlier. It is a neurological disease caused by a virus and affects the neurons controlling muscles. Some people recovered fully from the initial illness. Many had permanent disability with paralyses of limbs, but some were completely paralysed from head to foot and were placed in iron lungs as they could not breathe unaided. Those left with only partial paralysis were taught to ignore it and get on with their lives, which they most certainly did. Now, after many decades of overuse of muscles both strong and weak, they are suffering with PPS.

The problem is that all other causes of their symptoms must first be eliminated by various consultants, which takes a long time. I was eventually diagnosed with PPS. My right leg was originally affected and I could not walk for months, but it recovered. Now, at 76, the leg has again become weak. It makes walking difficult and my "good" arm has lots of wear to the ligaments due to overuse. A piece of bone has been removed from my shoulder to avoid the tendons and ligaments being worn through and causing paralysis of my good arm. My bicep has already ruptured and cannot be repaired.

At times my life has been very painful physically, but it never stopped me wanting to learn and achieve new things. When digital cameras became popular, I bought one that I could use with one hand and took a course in digital photography and editing photos. I really enjoyed repairing friends' pictures or even making them look a little more glamorous. I did a couple of "selfies" (as a self-portrait is now called), but when everyone kept asking who made me look so good I felt quite guilty. I didn't do it again after that as they obviously thought the camera was hiding a bad natural job! Such 'blows' were as naught, however, compared with my discovery in late November, 2005, of what real emotional pain felt like. First Rod, my husband of 47 years, was diagnosed with bowel cancer and told he had a month to live. He died two weeks later, shortly before I got to the hospital very early one morning. I was numb with shock. Five weeks earlier, he had been marshalling at a Brands Hatch motor race. He died on the day he was due to receive an award for 50 years' service as a flag marshal for the British Racing and Sports Car Club at their Annual Dinner on December 3, 2005.

I knew I must stand on my own two feet and get on with life, I never wanted to depend on my children, so I joined all the organisations locally that I could get to on foot or by bus (I was no longer driving due to my arm problems). I joined both the U3A, then a Sunday club, for talks followed by lunch, and a Friendship Group at the local hospital, who also met because they were alone on Sundays. I was invited by the local hospice to join their bereavement group and then I joined The Oddfellows (see **www.oddfellows.co.uk**), which is the organisation I have become most involved with. Through these groups, I made many friends and began to make a life for myself that has been very different from the married version. It was a busy life, yes, but I was still acutely aware of loneliness when I shut my door at night and was left all on my own. I wondered how I would cope with all the maintenance of my home. So far, with my trusty hammer, a set of screwdrivers and a can of WD40, I have managed most day-to-day repairs, but occasionally I have had to ask a kind neighbour to assist.

Four months after the death of my husband, I suffered a second emotional body blow when, after two-and-a-half years in the nursing home, my mother died at the age of 95. I was executor for both her and my husband and so I was now dealing with both estates. I refused to use a solicitor after one had negligently handled a will in which my mother had been a beneficiary. This had caused the firm of solicitors to be shut down by the Law Society and me to fight a very long battle on her behalf for her entitlement.

At a Friendship group meeting in September, 2007, I met Ralph Huntley, who was mourning his wife of 50 years. I asked him to join our table for lunch. He was an artist, as was his late wife. He told me his dream was to hold an exhibition of her wonderful work, but before that he had to clear their holiday home in Norfolk. They had spent many happy hours there painting the golden fields and wonderful trees of the peaceful landscapes. Two months later, he asked me out to dinner and we became firm friends.

I had a planned holiday to New Zealand and Australia with a neighbour, who had lost her husband shortly before mine died. She wanted company, so I volunteered to join her. While we were out there, Ralph phoned me and texted me at least twice a day. He also wrote letters to arrive at every hotel before I got there! He had fallen in love and couldn't wait for my return. I felt he had put me on a pedestal that I didn't deserve and my friends told me he was besotted. When I returned, I, too, fell in love with this very gentle and kind man. Alas, it was not to be one of the happiest times of my life. My children felt it was far too soon for me to be with another man – it was less than two years since their father had died. They didn't trust my judgment and felt I was at risk of being conned. We became estranged for many months and my sadness and isolation from them was extremely painful. I felt that as I was nearing 70 I had lived long enough to make my own decisions.

Time was not on our side and I knew we would both be happier living under the same roof. Ralph and I had found happiness together and relief from the loneliness that eats into your soul when you have lost a lifetime partner. We had faced the emptiness of our homes and the difficulty of making life purposeful again. For a while memories of the past were too painful to recall without tears. Together, we could cope by remembering and talking about our late partners and gradually putting back into our lives the joy shared with our former loved ones; we dwelt less in the dark place that loss can create.

Ralph had never left the UK, but I had travelled the world with Rod. My stories of the people and places I had been to made Ralph want to travel. At 75, he applied for his first passport and we went to Paris in the spring. We wandered by the Seine, sat in the Tuileries Gardens, ate out on the pavements, visited the Louvre and relaxed on a boat as we drifted past Notre Dame. The sun shone and time stood still - we were so happy together.

On our return we talked about Ralph's dream of an exhibition of his wife's work. I said I would help to plan it with him because I wanted to make his dream come true. Then, out of the blue one June day, he asked me to marry him. I wasn't sure it was the right thing to do as I knew it would be unpopular with my family. So I said I would think it over. Three weeks later, we were on a coach trip to Hereford on a sunny day with members of the bereavement group I had attended and I was looking at his profile against the window. He turned to me and smiled and I knew we were right together.

'I accept!' I said,

'Accept what?'

'I will marry you!' I laughed. His smile was as radiant as the sun.

'Oh! Bless you my love, I'll buy you an engagement ring tomorrow.'

'We won't tell everyone yet, I will just tell my friend Sylvia.'

Sylvia was sitting a few seats back. I whispered the news in her ear. She shrieked with joy and within seconds the whole coach knew we were engaged! Everyone seemed so happy for us, shouting their congratulations.

We planned our wedding for the beginning of October, 2008, in the little church where Ralph worshipped – All Souls Church in Crockenhill, Kent. I liked the people there. They had warmly welcomed me, even though I had been open about my atheism. I was still not sure the vicar would be prepared to marry us, but she came to Ralph's home to talk to us both and I explained my views.

"Why do you want to marry in church?" she asked.

"Because I feel the awe of the place and I want to feel my vows are taken seriously. It seems the right place to make such promises."

She seemed to accept that answer. She said had I answered that I was doing it for Ralph she would not have agreed to a church wedding. We actually discussed religion and faith very deeply and I discovered that she, too, had many doubts; we found we had much in common. My children and grandchildren initially said they would not attend the ceremony or reception, as they still felt I was wrong to remarry, but shortly beforehand they agreed to come to the church but not the reception. I felt extremely sad they could not be happy for me, but I was determined to enjoy my day. The wedding in October, 2008, was simple but the church was full when we married. Many members of the Bereavement Group came to share our joy and as the music rang out I knew I was doing the right thing. After our wedding, my children got to know Ralph better and finally they understood what he meant to me.

I told Ralph I would help him any way I could with arranging the exhibition of his late wife's art work. A year ahead of the event – planned for 4 weeks from 21 September -18 October 2009, - we booked Hall Place in Bexley, Kent, for the four-week memorial exhibition of Joan Marguerite Audrey

Huntley's very varied work. Early in 2009, we began reviewing the paintings together to decide which should be exhibited and which needed framing. I started to design cards of the paintings to sell for the local hospice; we were also cataloguing and pricing the drawings and paintings. By May, we had selected 79 pieces to be exhibited, many requiring framing within the next two months. Little did we know that once again our world was about to be shattered.

After visiting friends for a golden wedding lunch, Ralph was driving us home when he complained of a pain in his right side. It was so strong we had to pull over, but after walking about it stopped. I thought maybe the lunch had caused the problem. The pain kept recurring over the next few days and Ralph saw his GP. He had many tests over the next four months until in August he was diagnosed with terminal pancreatic cancer and only palliative care could be given. I asked the consultant how long he thought he would live.

"Possibly two months, but it is not an exact science," he replied. He described the worst-case scenarios while Ralph sat outside. I merely told him he would have chemotherapy. We had planned to steward the memorial exhibition ourselves, but Ralph was becoming too ill to carry on. Twenty-three people from the Friendship Group where we met offered their help as stewards. As Ralph became jaundiced, his chemotherapy was cancelled. He had both good and bad days, but increasingly I wondered if he would still be alive when the exhibition began. While he slept, I carried on with the cataloguing and pricing of all the pictures, handling the publicity, invitations to the private viewing day (September 21, 2009) and working out the stewards' rota.

I think I convinced him he was improving and that we would be able to get him to the exhibition in a wheelchair for the private viewing. He was certainly determined to be there on the opening day; he was even getting out of the wheelchair and walking around with a stick, talking to family and friends. The jaundice had made his face look brown and it was like a knife in my heart when everyone kept remarking how well he looked. I knew the truth, but I wanted this day to be his triumph in achieving his ambition for him and his late wife. I tried hard to melt into the background and just concentrate on the logistics. The exhibition was a great success and the money raised by the sale of the pictures went to both the hospice caring for Ralph and the "Stride For Life" campaign at the local hospital.

After the exhibition closed, Ralph's health rapidly deteriorated. Our daily life became full of visits by hospice nurses, community nurses and carers. He went into hospital for a stent to be fitted and this eased the jaundice for a while. After a fortnight in the hospice, on Christmas Eve, he was forced to leave. Social Services could not provide a care package over Christmas and as I was unable to lift Ralph or give him insulin injections for which both hands were needed. Social Services said he must go into a home. We were both in floods of tears as he tried to hug me, but they were adamant there was no alternative. We clung to each other and pleaded to let him stay until after Christmas, when his care package could be restored, but they refused.

Our Christmas Day in Ralph's room in the nursing home was spent talking about the joy of our love shared over the previous two years, the honeymoon on a cruise to Spain, the exhibition, and the fun times we had packed into our short time together. The day was very peaceful, providing some balm to the trauma of the enforced move. He died a month later in the home, six months from his diagnosis and 16 months from our wedding day. I had promised both Rod and Ralph they could die at home; my guilt and sadness are with me to this day, knowing that neither of the two men I had dearly loved had the peace of dying at home.

So once more I found myself a widow, alone in my home at 72. Could I start again, as I had done five years earlier? Even on the darkest days, a light sometimes shines. Just two days after Ralph died, I learnt that my first great-grandchild – a little girl, Rose, had been born to Bella and my Grandson Michael. When I looked into her tiny face, I knew life must go on and I must be part of it.

I also returned to the Bereavement Group. By talking and, surprisingly, laughing again with others who had lost their loved ones, my hopes grew that a way could be found to move forward again. No-one ever forgets, but there is a way to get through grief. For some, it takes years, if ever, but for others, like me, it is a realisation that you are still alive. You are sad, intensely so at times, but mourning constantly is destructive. By building something new for yourself or others, you can find happiness again. It may never be the happiness of a life before trauma, but I know life can have meaning again, with a positive outcome.

This was my experience; I found friendship beyond my expectations with David, my present partner. We met at the Bereavement Group. He told me he had lost both his wife of 53 years and his only child to cancer. She left two young children. We had a memorable first date at a lovely Italian Restaurant. I can't use peppermills, which need to be twisted with one hand while being held in the other, so David offered to do it for me. As he lifted it across the table, it knocked over the water carafe . . . which knocked over the bottle of wine . . . which poured into his dinner and ran across the table, pouring down my side to the floor! The waiters were most attentive and brought him another dinner after mopping up the mess of wine and water. I saw the funny side of it, but I did feel sorry for his embarrassment.

In the summer of 2010, I went to an Oddfellows business meeting and said I was now ready to start the daytime group that I had wanted to do before Ralph died. I arranged an inaugural tea party at a local cricket pavilion and 38 people attended. They were mostly from the groups I belonged to, while some were already Oddfellows. Nineteen people joined there and then. It is now going well. As Social Organiser, I arrange talks, outings, quizzes, games, lunches and charity events. Everyone who comes seems to thoroughly enjoy these events.

Another really enjoyable hobby for me since the 1990s has been learning all the intricacies of the computer. Of course, I am still learning! It changes so fast that I am finding it harder as I get older to keep up with each new invention, but my curiosity leads me to discover many new uses for my laptop. I've just got rid of my old PC. I've helped quite a few older people and have written little manuals to help them use their computers. It is never too late – us oldies just need TIME!

And there, Dear Reader, I must leave you – for the time being!

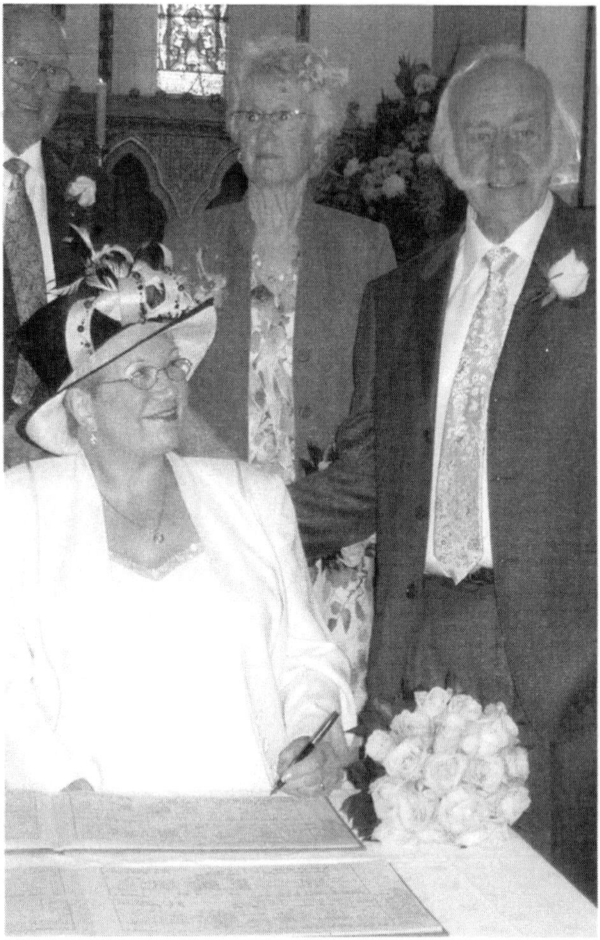

My Wedding to Ralph in 2008

ADDENDUMS

GRANDPARENTS

An incident that evoked strong feelings in my young life was the death of the only Grandfather I had known on 17 August 1946. My paternal Grandfather was a delightful gentleman who doted on me his only grandchild. He had fought in the Boer War and gained the South African Medal in 1901; it bears the bars 'Johannesburg', 'Paardenburg' and 'Cape Colony'. He was a boilermaker by trade; the noise in the workshops had burst his eardrums and he was absolutely stone deaf but he could lip read to a certain extent and always seems to have understood me. He had a shock of white hair and wore a thick tweedy jacket with leather patches on the elbows; he smelled leathery, perhaps because he always repaired the family shoes in the shed at the bottom of his garden, it also smelled of leather and glue. I loved watching Granddad at work in there, a tuneless whistle always came from his lips, it was more a sucking and blowing sound than a whistle really. I was happy to sit by him whilst he played cards with my father, the game was usually crib. Sometimes he would have a few sweets in his pockets and I had to guess which pocket they were in, his hand went into the pocket to feel whether my guess was correct but strangely I never seemed to get it right first time! I don't think I knew much about sleight of hand then.

Granddad could never hear the sirens or the bombs during the war because of his deafness and he preferred to stay in his own bed though Grandma did go in the shelter I think. On the night that the bomb dropped close to us the blast blew in his bedroom window sending shards of glass onto his bedding which left it shredded but by some miracle he was not hurt apart from a small cut on his forehead. I think the vibrations woke him but he did not realise what had happened until he put his feet out of bed onto the shards of broken glass.

One day my mother and father told me Granddad was very ill and we would be sleeping in my Grandparents house across the road from ours. My Grandparents bed had been bought downstairs into the front room where a weakling vigil began for the family watching over my dying Grandfather. It seems he had been playing bowls in the local recreation ground when he suffered a stroke. Nobody explained things to children in those days and the grown-ups whispered to each other in the presence of children thinking, quite wrongly, that a nine-year-old like me would not understand.

A day or two later the family discussed whether they should allow me to see my Granddad and they agreed to let me see him for a few minutes. I entered the room with my usual large bow of ribbon in my short hair, he seemed to recognise me immediately and smiled although he could not speak and his blue eyes twinkled in spite of his partial paralysis. I remember now his brown, weathered face against his white hair but most of all his smile, which, more than any words could say, told me he loved me. I think he knew when I kissed him that I loved him a great deal too. I hope he did for a few days later he died without my seeing him again. My first experience of death was very painful!

Granddad's wife, Edith, was a very religious woman of the Baptist faith. Her father had been a lay preacher and her life revolved around her churchgoing. On the thick brown wooden mantelshelf in what we would now call a living room, but was then called the kitchen, stood a big black marble clock. There was a canned fruit tin covered in wallpaper and filled with paper spills for fire lighting, a tin of pencils (one was always indelible), a letter holder and paper knife and two boxes for the church charities in which a few pennies were put each week. The room was furnished with a large heavy wooden table covered in a deep red chenille table cover. Underneath was a large bulbous legged stool covered in a piece of carpet on which I frequently sat at Grandma's knee; she sat in an upright wooden kitchen armchair with scrolled arms which I still have. When the housework was finished Grandma would knit or read books never allowing her hands to be idle except on Sunday's when no work was done and reading was limited to the Bible. Her knitting was prolific, frequently on four needles as she did all the socks and gloves for the whole family. I remember always needing elastic garters to hold up my socks but still they would concertina around my ankles.

Grandma's hair had never been cut as she considered it a sin in the eyes of God. Her clothes were generally black, grey or lilac with touches of lace at the front; two or three petticoats were worn beneath her dresses. Her clothes were covered by a cotton overall and a sacking apron in the mornings for heavy work and then she would wash and put on a cotton apron for the afternoon. When working she wore a Berlin wool cap, which was a tube, folded up at the bottom, sewn across the top with the corners sewn down like envelope flaps on either side. When she went out she always wore a hat and frequently a black and grey fox fur over her shoulders. I did not like the beady eyes in the head at all. Her handbag usually contained Fox's Glacier Mints or cough drops, one always being popped in her mouth before the church service began.

Grandma thought it was her duty to educate me in the word of the Lord and to encourage me to read the Bible. Although I was a keen pupil in many ways I could not accept the fact that when she did not know the answer to a question she always said it was 'God's Will which I should accept without question'. When something awful happened to people Grandma always said that it was because God had given us free will and sin was of our own making causing bad things to occur. But if all went well and something good happened it was always due to 'God's goodwill'; I always had the distinct impression that God took the kudos for the good and we lesser mortals got blamed for all the bad! My questioning of the virgin birth was tantamount to blasphemy in Grandma's eyes. But it was quite clear to me that Mary was pregnant before she married Joseph and if any girl had claimed an immaculate conception when unmarried when I was young I hardly think she would have been believed. I thought the people of Biblical times a bit gullible.

'How could it happen?' I would ask

'You really MUST NOT question the Good Lord,' she replied. I must have been a tiresome child to her at times with my endless questions but her exasperation was generally limited to a heavy sigh, her self control being as strong as the corsets that held her figure upright.

However, like all children in the 1940/50s I attended Sunday school and was indoctrinated by their teaching and Grandma's persistence and I became a very religious teenager.

I always felt I could chat to Grandma and I suppose in many ways she was my mentor. She certainly made a lasting impression on me and strangely I have always felt she was nearer to me after her death than many other of my family who have since died. In my teens I accompanied her to evening service in the local Baptist Church though I often found that the services were boring and found myself counting the bricks on the back wall there.

I also attended the local Mission Church joining a group called The Christian Endeavour; I think part of the attraction was a lad with flaming red hair whom I really fancied! However my feelings were totally unrequited! My father insisted I left the Mission when gossip did the rounds about a young woman from the Bible class who tried to commit suicide by gassing herself in a room at the back of the church because she had fallen in love with the married minister who preached there.

Whether he reciprocated or not I have no idea but my father said there was no smoke without fire and I was consequently banned from that establishment.

My maternal widowed Grandmother lived next door to my family, she was a plump cuddly lady, very industrious about the house, a peacemaker, very witty, constantly washing curtains and chair covers. She crocheted doilies, blankets, bags and even brooches on which she sewed glass beads for presents. She sang hymns while she worked but her especial favourite was 'What a Friend we Have in Jesus' sung while she scrubbed the washing on a washboard in a galvanised iron bath which caused her voice to wobble up and down as the Sunlight soap was rubbed into the clothes. Another favourite was 'Daisy, Daisy Give Me Your Answer Do'. I think of her on washing day standing in the scullery with the washing bath sitting on top of planks of wood covering the bath the family used to bathe in. The vitreous enamel bath was under the kitchen window with the foot end tucked under the big white butler sink. The wooden planks over the bath were covered in either lino or oilcloth and this was used as a work surface for preparing all the food. There were no taps on the bath, water was heated in a large free-standing electric boiler from which buckets were filled and the hot water was then tipped into the bath. A bit of hose-pipe was used from the sink tap to add cold water. Bath water was generally shared by at least two members of a family, the least dirty bathing first.

My maternal Grandmother had 13 grandchildren all of whom were made welcome and fed with mountains of food, lots of jam tarts, stodgy puddings and cups of coca or home made ginger beer. Stews with heaps of potatoes were also a favourite. She always pronounced stew as 'stoo' and Tuesday as 'Toosday'.

Between my maternal Grandmother's back yard and that of my parents was a high wooden fence; on Grandma's side was a small ladder. Her head would pop over the top of the fence and she would call for my mother, however names seemed to elude her on most occasions and in consequence she shouted all her four daughters names 'Daisy, Edie, Violet, Ivy!' which seemed effective.

Sometimes Grandma gave her grandchildren a 'Thruppeny' piece as 3d was pronounced in those days. We looked forward to this little bit of pocket money but as sweets were rationed it was mostly spent on other things. I bought crest china at jumble sales sometimes.

One day Grandma took one of my cousins and me on the 'Daffodil' steamer to Southend for the day, which was a huge treat at that time, the equivalent of a trip to Disneyland in 1996! We were very,

very excited because we could not have holidays during the war and afterwards our parents had very little money.

I loved Grandma, though I thought she had some very odd habits like cleaning her ears with hairpins and making odd noised in her throat. If I stayed with her at night in her big, squishy feather bed she would take off her corsets before putting on her voluminous nightie then she would scratch her middle making happy noises of relief. If she passed wind she never said 'Pardon me'; it was always 'MANNERS' in a loud voice. She delighted in food, whist drives, cream slices and a nice cup of tea. Her working life in service had begun for half days when she was eleven years old and became full time at thirteen years. It was a hard life working for a woman who had very naughty twin sons. If they broke something they blamed my Grandmother and their mother invariably believed them.

Grandma died aged 72 when I was sixteen years old after my mother and I had nursed her through three strokes over a period of nine months. I have never forgotten these months; they were good training for later years when I had elderly relatives to care for. My Grandmother was the first dead person that I had seen. I see her dead face now looking like white marble, her jaw bandaged to her head. No lines just an unrecognisable face, she no longer looked like my wrinkled, smiley Grandma.

EPILOGUE

Polio peaked between the 1920s and the early 1960s. Mercifully, it has been almost eradicated in the western world since the first vaccine was introduced in the 1950s. Consequently, however, the disease is no longer feared and has become almost forgotten. Most of us feel great sympathy when we see young people with beautiful faces suffering dreadful diseases, but please think of those whose physical beauty is no longer there and who need constant care and support. Many people were affected by polio - small children ... people in the armed forces during the Second World War, whose fighting was ended by the paralysis . . . teenagers . . . mothers with young children they might never hold in their arms again. Pre-vaccine, the disease could strike anyone, rich or poor; it spread indiscriminately.

Polio can affect just a group of muscles controlling a limb - or it can totally paralyse someone, in which case they may no longer be able to breathe without artificial means. When victims recovered from the initial stages of the disease, they made intense efforts to work the remaining 'good' muscles over many years. This has now taken its toll. Many are suffering renewed paralysis and increasing weakness; many who recovered enough to walk are now losing that ability once more. Where this is affecting their lungs, there is the additional problem of breathing difficulties. Arms and hands are becoming too weak to do all the things they were able to do before. The early symptoms seem to be reappearing and are exacerbated by old age. This book is dedicated to all those people now suffering the severe effects of Post Polio Syndrome.

If you would like to help please donate to: **The British Polio Fellowship, Citibase, 44 Clarendon Road, Watford, Hertfordshire, WD17 1JJ.**

Freephone 0800 043 1935 Main Switchboard: 01923 312 400

The British Polio Fellowship has a network of branches around Britain for the support and care of polio victims. Head Office also produces a magazine which educates and informs members about a wide range of topics concerning them.:

Email: info@britishpolio.org.uk **Website:** www.britishpolio.org.uk

"The British Polio Fellowship-N. W. Kent District' like many branches is really struggling to provide outings and events for their many seriously disabled members. Transport day ambulances can take only very limited numbers of wheelchairs to provide outings and they are extremely expensive.

by Barbara Blackston Huntley

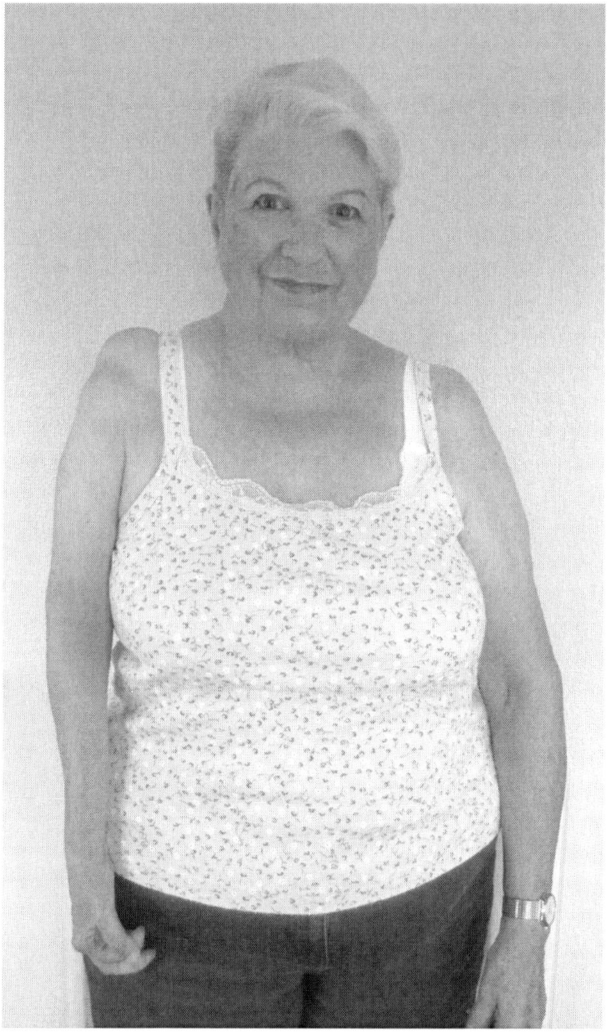

The Author – Barbara Blackston Huntley

Forgive Me For Not Shaking Hands